GW00578135

Ordering Information:
Special discounts are available on quantity purchases by yoga
studios, conferences and festivals. Contact erin@aquinyoga.
com for more information.
publisher at the address above.

Published by Emergence Education Press

ISBN-10:0-9969285-5-3
ISBN-13:978-0-9969285-5-7

For Audrey and Steve
Thank you for making this life a wild and
wonderful journey.

Acknowledgements

There are so many people who have contributed to this project in some way. Since I first stepped on a yoga mat nearly two decades ago I have learned about yoga from countless instructors and students. In Chinese Medicine school, I was fortunate enough to work with incredible teachers and peers and to thank them all properly would fill up the pages of this book before it begins. There are a few people however who were directly involved with making this book come to life that I must extend my gratitude towards.

To my wild child Audrey Ray, I wrote most of this book in the pockets of the first year of your life. Thank you for being my muse and connecting me to love and devotion like no one else could.

Steve Haase, you were not only moral support during this project, but also photographer, editor, first reader, dinner chef, baby whisperer, cheerleader, latte-maker, marketing guru, website doctor and the most amazing husband and friend I could ever hope for. Thank you.

To my parents John and Julie Aquin and my Nana Julie, thank you for raising me with open hearts and minds and giving me the freedom to discover the spiritual path in the many forms that may take.

A warm thank you to Jeff Carreira and Amy Edelstein for not only cheering me on but for honouring me with the offer to publish this book.

Special thanks to the team of people who touched this book: Rebecca Mullen my coach and Allison Mecham Evans my inspiring writing pal. I learned so much from both of you. Thank you to Laura Didyk for editing much of the book, Jon Haase for editing the photos and Steve Deckert for hooking us up with a very fine camera.

~Contents~

Introduction:
My Unexpected Discovery   1

Awakening the Heart: An Elemental Fairytale   3

Preparing for Your Journey Through the Elements   8

The Elements:
Water   21

Fire   41

Wood   61

Metal   81

Earth   101

Elemental Asanas:
Before You Begin   123

Water Poses   133

Fire Poses   141

Wood Poses   147

Metal Poses   154

Earth Poses   160

A Sample Elemental Yin Yang Practice   168

Resources   169

My Unexpected Discovery

When I began studying Chinese Medicine over a decade ago, I expected to find ways of helping people live with greater overall health and well-being. Using acupuncture and herbs as part of a holistic treatment plan, I saw firsthand how this medicine could coax the physical body into improved health by correcting its energetic flow and unblocking stagnation built up by years of stress and neglect. At the time, I had already been teaching yoga for a few years and hoped this new field of study would provide me with tools to help my students and clients even more. Chinese Medicine was one step along the road to reshaping their lives by working in closer alignment with the cycles of nature.

What I did not expect was that the medicine would rewire my thinking on everything from health to my own yogic path. Over the years, my time on the yoga mat had evolved from being part spiritual, part physical practice into a profound metaphorical path and mirror for life. While much of my education in Chinese Medicine was focused on hunting down different pathological patterns and fixing problems of the body and mind, there was a richness and beauty in the philosophy and I fell in love with it.

While I have always appreciated the classical yogic texts, the principles of the yamas and niyamas, as well as allegorical guides like the Bhagavad Gita, I don't relate to them in a way that has been personally transformative. What does resonate is the philosophy of Yin-Yang and the Five Elements. The idea that the natural world provides symbols that we can use to understand and navigate life makes sense to me. As a clinical practitioner the insights and wisdom of Chinese Medicine started to seep out onto my mat and into my classes.

Over the course of nearly fifteen years, teaching thousands of classes, I developed a unique form of yoga inspired by the wisdom of Chinese Medicine: Elemental Yin Yang Yoga. This style of yoga is the best of two asana worlds, blending challenging flow postures (Yang) followed by a sequence of long-held more passive poses (Yin). The A-type yoga student who craves vigorous physicality in their practice will find it in the Yang flow and will also experience postures that challenge them to be still for longer periods of time and relax deeply during the Yin portion of class. The yogi who loves a slow pace and resists breaking a sweat will be rewarded in the Yin sequence after exploring the more dynamic, energetic Yang flow.

If you are a yoga practitioner or a teacher who wants to find deeper meaning in your practice, this book will help you take the themes you find most powerful from this system out into your world.

Elemental Yin Yang Yoga is a lifestyle practice that begins on the mat and expands to touch all aspects of your life, from your work to your intimate relationships. Please enjoy this dynamic exploration and may it fuel your yoga journey.

~Erin Aquin
www.aquinyoga.com

Awakening the Heart: An Elemental Fairytale

It is the first day of spring but snow still covers the fields, forests, and cities without discrimination. This icy blanket has prevented most citizens from working today, but in the central palace the top officials have gathered, ready to discuss the state of the Empire they serve. The winter has been hard on everyone and each member of the government is here to plead their case to the Prime Minister in hopes of the resources they need to repair and rebuild.

The Head of Transportation is a plump, disheveled man who grumbles about how far he has travelled to be here along broken roads. Next to him sits the official in charge of power, a rather unscrupulous man who interrupts, pulling focus to his cause.

"The roads are in near perfect condition compared to the state of the power plant. I must insist that our priority for this spring be to strengthen infrastructure for my department. This winter we experienced rolling blackouts constantly. It is a wonder these outages haven't caused panic or death! We cannot sustain consistent power throughout the empire unless we receive a sizable boost in funding right away."

The Irrigation Official sneers and the officials in charge of agriculture and food processing lock eyes. They have prepared a more ingratiating approach.

"Prime Minister, we know you have many options to consider for how to allocate our spring resources. You always make the right decision and we are so grateful that you consider everyone's needs equally. We hope that any extra resources will continue to be shared with our department. Not only do we have repairs to make to avoid more damage from spring floods but we need to invest in the newest agricultural tools in order to get the most out of this year's harvest. While roads and the power grid are important, without nutrients our people will starve."

The weathered-looking General explodes "Your groveling is disgraceful! Who cares about roads and expensive equipment at a time like this? Prime Minister, we need to secure our borders right away. Our enemies surround us and get bolder by the day. If we don't show our strength, there won't be any land left to care for!"

At this, the meeting dissolves into chaos. The Prime Minister's face goes pale and falls into his hands. He tries to call everyone back to order but his voice is too weak. While he technically holds the organizational power to delegate and decide who should get what and how to proceed, the truth is the resources these officials are tripping over themselves to obtain simply do not exist. For years it has been his private secret: the nation has been operating over budget, falling deeper and deeper into debt and now its time has run out.

Suddenly the door flies open. A petite, striking woman enters and all heads turn to gaze at her. A thick silence settles over the room interrupted only by the clicking of the woman's shoes against the marble floor. The newest arrival is known to all as the personal Receptionist of the Empress. She is the gatekeeper of the Inner Chamber, deciding who is given the honour of meeting with the figurehead of the nation. For years this has been offered to no one. The Receptionist also has a reputation for her skill in the ways of alchemy.

"Greetings esteemed officials, the Empress has arrived to join your meeting."

She makes a quick inspection of the room and when satisfied, she opens the doors fully. A radiant woman dressed in elegant robes gracefully floats in and begins to make her way towards her seat at the table. She is flanked by her most loyal and fearsome companion, her personal guard. The officials are awestruck and they bow in reverence of their Empress. She takes her seat and everyone else follows.

The Prime Minister is the first to speak. "We wish to welcome Your Imperial Majesty to this meeting."
She nods her head in acknowledgment.
"We have been discussing how best to deal with the various needs of the different sectors and departments as we move into spring. Each official has asked for more resources to support their work."

"What a very difficult problem for you, dear Prime Minister" she replies sweetly. "And have you told these esteemed officials the truth of the matter?"
The Prime Minister's face falls once again. "No, Your Imperial Majesty."
"Ah. Well, the truth is, we have no resources left," she says plainly.

"You are all aware that I have been absent from public life due to a heartbreak I do not wish to discuss. For the past few years our dear Prime Minister has had to perform both his duties and mine. As wonderful a leader as he is, our roles are very different. As Empress, it is my duty to guide all of you and share my divine vision. Until now, my lack of involvement has forced you all to take on more than you can possibly care for, and I vow to you all that starting on this day, I will be the Empress you deserve."

The unprecedented humility with which she speaks is moving.
"I have hidden myself away for too long," she continues, "and in the midst of my own suffering have allowed our empire to suffer. While I cannot heal or undo the damage that has been done, my hope is that all of us working harmoniously together can cultivate the strength and vitality our nation needs to prosper."

After a few moments the Prime Minister breaks the sacred silence following the announcement by the Empress.
"Your Imperial Majesty, I think I speak for everyone when I say we are all moved and honoured by your words. With all due respect, knowing that our resources are severely depleted and all of the departments under your rule are in need of immediate funding, how shall we proceed?"
At this, the alchemist steps forward to stand beside her Empress.
"Thank you for this observation and for your important question," she says playfully, with a hint of sarcasm.

"As you may be aware I am skilled in the alchemical arts. Our Gracious Imperial Majesty has given me a special ritual to begin the cultivation process needed to revitalize our resources. It will take time for the transformation to be visible, but I have already begun practicing special movements and meditations that I will soon teach to all of you."

"I don't understand," says the general, "How can a ritual of movements and meditations create the practical resources we need to fuel the empire?"

The Empress smiles, then says, "Do you doubt that your inner attitude influences the way you express yourself in the world? It may sound like child's play for the uninitiated, but the rituals my alchemist speaks of are also practical in nature, requiring discipline and awareness. In time, with regular practice, you will become more aware of just how important your work is. Once you have allowed your inner compass to be recalibrated you will stop wasting your precious time and energy on things that work against you. I have had a vision of the glorious destiny of our Empire. But no destiny is guaranteed. It will take all of us working together in harmony to fulfill our highest purpose as a united body. This ritual will just be the first step on the journey."

The Officials are the vital organs and they bow to their Empress (the Heart) ready to perform their specialized functions so the Empire (the body and mind) may flourish. The mysterious ritual begins at the top of a yoga mat with the sound of OM…

Preparing for Your Journey Through The Elements

Chinese Medicine and the philosophy that supports it has evolved over thousands of years. Countless books have been written on the practice and theory of Yin Yang (rhymes with song) and the Five Elements, yet the jewels contained within this body of knowledge are relatively unknown in the yoga world. Interestingly, there are similarities between some core yoga theory and Chinese philosophy. Although the passage of information may have been nonexistent between these two fields of study, both include an explanation of life-force energy: prana in yoga and qi/essence in Chinese Medicine.

As you embark on this journey you will find more similarities between the two systems and learn how to apply this wisdom both on and off your yoga mat. This book will be your guide and the first humble footholds on the path of study and personal investigation.

Before you can get a clear sense of this style of yoga, you need to understand the basics. It may take time for these concepts to become familiar to you, but if you open yourself to viewing the world through this lens you will soon grasp how the ancient philosophers and yogis saw the natural world and why much of that perspective is useful even in our current time. Before we jump in let's get prepared for the journey by getting acquainted with some of the key concepts and terms that you will see over and over again throughout the book.

Dao & Enlightenment

Questioning how existence came to be and the purpose of life are often at the heart of why any practitioner sets out on the spiritual path. All the religions and spiritual traditions of the world attempt to answer these big questions or at the very least provide a framework for deeper inquiry.

Your being drawn to Elemental Yin Yang Yoga is no different and likely began with an internal pull for you to spend time on your yoga mat. At first you may have felt the call to practice because you heard it was good for you or would offer a pleasant break in your hectic life. If you continued with any consistency, you may have noticed your less savoury habits and thoughts lost their power over you. Or perhaps you had an experience related to yoga so undeniably transformative that it has since catalyzed a major life change. And yet, when you try to explain your experience, words fall flat in comparison to the enormity of the wholeness and wonder you have seen.

In Chinese philosophy, the unnamable, pre-cognitive power or energy you feel in those deep moments of transformation is pointing you towards what the famous Chinese philosopher Lao Tzu called the Dao. Through his text the Dao de Jing, Lao Tzu poetically attempts to point at that which is beyond the knowing of the mind. The unknowable, non-dual, wholeness that came before our physical universe.

Meditators and yogis alike refer to this state of no-separation as "enlightenment" and many spend their lives devoted to peeling away layers of hardwired thinking in hopes of witnessing it, even for a moment. It is no wonder that the concept of Dao is the most elusive in Chinese philosophy—something you can attempt to locate with lyrical language but which can't be fully articulated or held by the rational mind.

"Tao (Dao) existed before words and names, before heaven and earth, before the ten thousand things. It is the unlimited father and mother of all limited things."
~The Tao Te Ching of Lao Tzu (translation by Brian Browne Walker)

Yin and Yang

In Chinese Philosophy the Dao gives rise to yin and yang. Everything in our Universe is made up of yin and yang and can be defined by this relationship. To understand these two energies, let us first examine the tai ji, the universal symbol outlined by a circle.

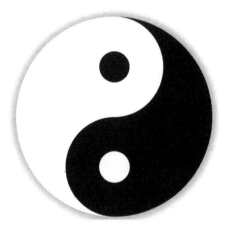

The darker side of the circle represents yin. It is cool in nature, moves downward and corresponds to the interior structures of the body like the bones and blood. The lighter side of the circle is symbolic of yang. It is warmer than yin, moves upwards and is symbolic of the exterior layers of muscle and skin in the body. The first type of relationship that yin and yang have, and the easiest to understand, is one of opposition. Their opposition does not exist in separation or discord from the other, but rather as "two sides of the same coin" in a state of a dynamic interplay.

Just as the process of homeostasis keeps stability in the body by making constant adjustments to the physiological functions in our body, yin and yang are always adjusting and compromising based on feedback from the other. They are two personalities of the same energy.

Next, notice that the darker yin half contains a spot of light and the lighter yang half hosts a spot of dark. The next relationship that yin and yang share are not as two absolute concepts but as relative partners who always contain a fragment of the other. A summer day is yang (warm) compared to a winter day, but more yin (cool) than the heat found at the centre of an active volcano. Both are considered hot, but when compared to one another there is a spectrum of relativity. Yin and yang can only be defined in a relative relationship and one can not exist without the other.

In the body for instance, even with all its internal structures (more yin in nature) perfectly in place it would be lifeless without yang's energy making physiological functions happen. The structure of the lungs is yin but the act of breathing is yang. Yin depends on yang for movement and yang has no home without yin.

Finally the symbol appears to have a tail of yang seeping into Yin and vice versa. Just as day gives way to night and night fades into day, the dance of these two energies reminds us that nothing in life is a constant. Someone who pushes themselves to the limit staying awake for several days to finish a project will eventually burn out and need quality rest in order to recover. We can't live in only one half of the circle. Summer must give way to fall and fall to winter in order for new growth to occur in the spring.

Quick Reference Chart

Yin	Yang
Cooler	Warmer
Interior	Exterior
Lower	Upper
Night	Day
Structures of the Body	Functions of the Body
Winter	Summer
Water	Fire
Long-held yoga postures	Fast-paced yoga flows

Yin Yang Breakdown

The concepts of yin and yang can be challenging to work with at first since our thinking often tricks us into believing that our physical world is made up of solid things rather than energy particles. Even something that we classify as "yin" contains its fair share of designated yang energy. For instance, if you observe a yogi in Savasana (Corpse pose), the most yin pose of all time, you will see that while the practitioner is lying still, making no muscular or voluntary effort at all, below the surface, yang energy is keeping the yogi's important life-giving functions going. The yogi is involuntarily breathing while the heart circulates blood throughout the body, and the digestive organs do their thing—the body is a bustling hub of Yang energy despite the peace and relaxation the yogi is drifting in.

To help you understand Yin and Yang more deeply in your yoga practice, break the following postures down into their Yin and Yang aspects and see if you can break them down even one level further.

Mountain Pose
Triangle Pose
Crow Pose
Reclined Twist

Applying Wisdom on the Mat

Introducing the concepts of yin-yang and the Five Elements makes this style of yoga unlike any other. Through Elemental Yin Yang Yoga, you will begin to understand and appreciate the cycles of nature and life more deeply. Working with the Five Elements closely on the mat will not only enhance your yoga practice, but the elements themselves will come to act as powerful metaphors for your life in ways that will enhance and expand your creativity and perspective (Wood), connection and love (Fire), wisdom and will power (Water), insight and inspiration (Metal), and your capacity to nourish yourself and the world (Earth).

The physical yoga practice acts like a ritual that bridges your intellectual understanding with symbols that speak the language of the subconscious. Together these pieces provide a launch pad for greater personal well-being, self-knowledge and the management of Qi.

Qi

In yoga theory a central feature that differentiates physical asana from other forms of exercise is working with "prana," or life-force energy. Closely linked to the act of breathing, this essential substance is what animates us on and off the mat. In Elemental Yin Yang Yoga the vital life-force energy is called Qi (pronounced "chi"). Qi is the unseen power that courses through the energetic meridians of the body and although it has some subtle differences with prana, it's similar enough that the two terms can be used, more or less, synonymously.

Congenital Qi

We each begin life with varying amounts of Qi. Think of this as a trust fund you are given at birth, but instead of money, the account holds your genetic makeup and a reserve of Qi given to you by your parents. Some people are born with a huge amount of this type of Qi in the bank and can stretch it into old age. Others come into the world with very little of this Congenital Qi and lacking a solid head start, must rely heavily on a different kind of Qi to fuel them.

Acquired Qi

Acquired Qi is energy one gets from eating and drinking. Unlike the trust-fund of Congenital Qi, it can be replenished. In order to get high quality Qi in abundance, a healthy lifestyle, adequate nutrition, and a properly functional digestive system is required. If someone is lacking in one of these areas, it will hinder their ability to garner enough Acquired Qi and they will more quickly deplete their reserves of Congenital Qi.

Yoga is a practice of learning how to cultivate and manage both types of Qi. While any physical practice takes a certain amount of energy to perform, an ideal yoga program flushes the meridians of stress and stagnation, allowing blockages to be resolved. It also helps to fortify the digestive system and redirect overflowing Qi from one area to another that needs it more. Yoga is a powerful method that can assist you not only in building Qi, but in conserving it by learning to output only that which is needed and no more.

Exploring the Elements

To help you navigate through the elements I have provided you with touchstones through each chapter. Most are self-explanatory but in case you decide not to read the book front to back but instead create your own path, a few words need to be said about some of the fundamentals you will see repeated throughout the book.

The Organs

Without being a Chinese Medicine diagnostician, the patterns and functions of the organs for each of the Five Elements throughout the book may seem strange and incorrect to you. Therefore it is important to remember that while we may use the words "heart," "kidney," "lung," "liver," etc., the functions I share with you may not apply to what you know scientifically.

Think of the organs instead as a way Chinese Medicine groups certain functions and patterns and not as a hard and fast rule of how the physiological structures work in the body. If you are interested in learning more about the similarities and differences between the Chinese and Western models of the body, check out the resource section at the back of this book to expand your understanding.

Constitution—The Element of Primary Influence

The chapters on the Five Elements contain a wide range of information including several symbols and themes relevant for Elemental Yin Yang yogis. One association you may be less familiar with is the idea of constitution. While there are very detailed explanations on the formation and function of the element most influential to each individual according to Chinese Medicine, for our purposes you can think of constitution simply as the filter and lens through which you experience the world. Just as a coloured lens obscures the images before you and a filter removes some of the raw input it receives, your constitution applies its own tint and sifts experiences to suit its assumptions and limitations.

Constitution Is Not an Excuse

One of the most accessible ways to get to know the Five Elements is in relationship to other individuals. When you can take a bundle of qualities and symbols and trace those patterns back to people you know it is easier to relate to the element more in its human form. However, in Chinese medicine being able to identify a person's constitutional makeup with any accuracy takes years.

In my yoga teacher trainings the most popular question I am asked after sharing this information is:

"What is my constitution?"

While I may have an idea about the questioner's primary element of influence after spending some time with them, I always hesitate to give a direct answer.

Over the years I have heard too many people use their constitutional diagnosis in various schools of medicine, such as the Indian system of Ayurveda to pigeon-hole themselves or others. I have a particular aversion to people who say "I can't help getting angry because I am a Wood type" or "I don't like vigorous exercise because I am too Earthy and Kapha."

In one Five Element class I attended the instructor showed his clinical skills by sharing his ideas about the constitution of each student in the class. In one exchange, he said to a student:

"Your primary element is Metal."

"No, my constitution is Wood," she replied.

They went back and forth for a few minutes, the teacher pointing out the students "Metal" qualities and the student arguing why she was a "Wood" type (by the way, Wood people tend to get angry as a first defense and this student seemed to jump right into being argumentative before hearing the instructor out). The conversation went on for a while and after the class the student was visibly upset.

"How can he think that about me?!" she said almost in tears. "And what if he is right? What if I have been living as Wood all this time but really I am Metal?!"
It was clear that somewhere in this student's education, she came to believe that one constitution is better than another.

It may sound ridiculous, but after learning about these personalities, people may develop strong attachments and aversions to the Five Elements and also have a deep need to know what category they fit into in order to know who they are. Knowing your constitution isn't license to act poorly or accentuate the worst qualities of that element. There is no optimal constitution since each have their strengths and weaknesses and depend heavily on the person who is expressing those traits.

Why Think About Constitution At All?

At this point in history we don't need more ways to categorize and compartmentalize ourselves or one another. Far too many people cling tightly to a diagnosis and use that to paralyze themselves from developing further. For that reason, it is important to remember that the examples of constitution in this book are merely tools to highlight one point on the wide spectrum of possibilities for how a particular element will be expressed in human beings. Circumstances such as culture, religion, education, gender identification, and so much more, go into the make-up of a person. Constitution is just one of the many complex ways we can relate to others.

The reason this information is useful is because it teaches you more about the nature of the Five Elements and offers an idea of how they may express themselves in your human relationships. As a former clinician, understanding what element most influenced the patient in front of me would impact how I spoke to them and treated them. An Earth type might require a more supportive and nurturing attitude from me in order to change a harmful health habit like eating junk food. A Wood type on the other hand may need a firm "big picture" view of what the consequences could be if they don't change their ways.

I urge you to use the constitutional information with care and remember that while constitution may include your greatest weakness it also includes your greatest strength.

The Big Picture

We are at a crux in our human story that begs for more people who are aware, awake, and connected to a desire to make positive changes for our global community. While it may be a stretch to believe that a regular yoga practice can change the world, it is highly likely that a practice with a focused intention can change you personally. The yin part of the practice invites you into sacred stillness even in the face of discomfort, boredom, or displeasure in your own skin. The yang portion of this discipline invites you to discover your full power and question your assumptions about what is and is not possible in the present moment. These two energies combined teach you how to both work hard and let go, to play and relax so that you have the capacity to be a positive force in a world that desperately needs you.

Get Free Videos, Audios and Elemental Resources
Visit: www.aquinyoga.com/elemental

Water

"Water does not resist. Water flows. When you plunge your hand into it, all you feel is a caress. Water is not a solid wall, it will not stop you. But water always goes where it wants to go, and nothing in the end can stand against it. Water is patient. Dripping water wears away a stone. Remember that, my child. Remember you are half water. If you can't go through an obstacle, go around it. Water does."
~ **Margaret Atwood,** *The Penelopiad*

The Dive

I stand shoulder deep in the ocean. Even though the water is not cold and I am wearing a wetsuit, I can feel a chill in my bones, or maybe it is the fear. My partner Steve looks at me and asks, "Are you sure you are okay to do this?"
I shoot back a smile, one I know he can see right through, and say, "Totally."

Steve and I are being led on this adventure by our kind scuba instructor Rachel. She spends the next few minutes going over the important things one last time. We review the hand signals we should use in order to communicate, how to equalize our ears to deal with the pressure underwater, how to locate the regulator (the mouthpiece that helps you breathe), and, in the rare event that the mouthpiece slips out, how to get rid of any water that collects inside of it. I flub my way through this final lesson as I'm being knocked around by the waves. My face must reveal my true feelings because Rachel makes a point to assure me she will be with us the whole time. Intellectually, I believe her, but fear has gripped me and assures me that it too will be my constant companion on this adventure.

As we start to walk deeper into the rough water, panic rises to a new height within me. I feel claustrophobic in the mask but now we are starting to descend and I can't remember the hand signal for: "I am freaking out!"

I do, however, remember not to swim with wide arm strokes but instead use my feet like flippers. Steve apparently forgets this instruction and as he swims by he rips the regulator out of my mouth. Without noticing, he continues forward and I am left floating underwater at the back of our group. Suddenly, the tool delivering me breath and life is floating beside me. I hear Rachel's voice singing in my head: "If you lose it, just locate your regulator and put it back in your mouth. Suck your cheeks in and blow the out the water. Breathe and continue your dive."

I test out her instructions with everything at stake and miraculously feel the air return to my desperate lungs. After successfully managing this problem, my fear begins to dissolve. For the next hour underwater, our little team is weightless with nothing but the sound of our breathing and the unbelievable beauty of ocean life. On our dive that day we meet schools of colourful fish, a tiny octopus, and several sea turtles that swim between us and the sunshine above. We even encounter a few sharks swimming in their cave. I am so lost in the magic of the experience that Rachel has to monitor the levels of underwater "air" I have left. When another check tells her I am getting low on resources we head back up to the surface.

Crossing the threshold of the unknown into this new world is nothing short of magical. The life happening below the surface of the ocean is vast and holds mysteries and curiosities that as a land dweller I could not have imagined before experiencing it. The fear I had going into my first dive was real and valid, but I am grateful that, in this instance, I found a way forward with the help of people that had the wisdom of experience to guide me into the wonder that awaited me below the surface.

Water

Water is a precious resource that supports life. This element not only covers more than 70 percent of Earth's surface but makes up more than half of the average human body. While we depend on water to sustain us, water can destroy as much as it can create. Rain can flood low-lying geographical sectors, rivers can swell beyond their usual boundaries and a tsunami can wipe out an unlucky area in a matter of minutes. In Chinese philosophy Water represents our inner essence and personal resources. It is the wisdom that lies beyond the unknown. It is the flowing nature of life, the chill of winter and cloak of darkness, an element to be revered and never underestimated.

The Season of Water: Winter

Winter is a time for regeneration. On the surface the season may appear to be nothing more than a bleak expanse of time along the wheel of the year that many of us hide from inside temperature-controlled homes. Yet winter is, of course, necessary for many plants and animals. During these cold months, the earth sleeps wrapped in its blanket of snow. Both plants and hibernating animals conserve their energy until it is time to reemerge in the spring. Yet in the midst of this more dormant phase, the blueprint for the year ahead is held in the seeds below ground. Like a human egg, seeds if given the right circumstances can grow to their full potential into the plant they are meant to be, and winter is an important part of that preparation and gestation period.

Of all the seasons, winter is the most yin in nature because it is the coldest and darkest. This turn of the wheel invites the yogi to engage in self-reflective practices, such as meditation and Yin Yoga, and to practice conservation on and off the yoga mat.

In places that host drastically cold and dark winters, practicing yoga in heated rooms can bring comfort and a respite from chilly temperature. This is the perfect time for yogis to accept winter's invitation to slow down, reflect, and regenerate in the shadow of short days and long nights.

The Organs

Water is represented in the body by the Kidneys (more often called the singular "Kidney" in Chinese Medicine) and the Bladder.

Water Yin: The Kidney - The Power Official

The Kidneys in Chinese medicine help form the basis of life. While in Western Medicine the main function of this organ pair is to remove waste from the blood and transfer it for elimination with excess water further down the urinary system, Chinese Medicine assigns this organ other essential roles that have nothing to do with the actual physiological function.

In our Elemental fairytale the Kidney is the power official. This official is in charge of harnessing the raw power of the wild river and diverting it towards a central dam in order to be concentrated into useable energy for the empire. In the body this potential power is processed into the ingredients needed for Yin Yang, qi and stores our most essential fluids. Kidney energy is needed at all stages of life, beginning with development in the womb, continuing with childhood growth and sexual maturity, all the way into old age. Without adequate and appropriate levels of Kidney qi and essence, dysfunction can more easily take root.

Kidney problems can have drastic consequences. During rolling blackouts, already weakened infrastructure becomes more vulnerable as security systems fail and hospitals lack the life-giving ability of equipment that runs off the power grid. When you lack adequate power, even the most stable and efficient parts of your body and mind will be thrown into chaos if it continues over time.

Healthy Kidneys and flourishing Water energy ensure that the basis of yin and yang energy is protected and not wasted or used frivolously.

Water Yang: The Bladder - The Official of the Wastewater Reservoir

While the Kidney(s) is yin and stores the vital essence required to fuel the body, the Bladder is yang and acts more like a portal, constantly being filled and emptied so that wastewater doesn't back up and flood the system.

The main power station is governed by the Kidney(s) and is of central importance in the energy system of the Empire but it needs this outlet to manage waste water. The Bladder assists in making sure the system doesn't become overloaded or experience a backwards flowing of impure fluid. Both physically and energetically the Bladder assists in flushing leftover resources that are no longer useful so that they don't bog down or burden us.

Themes of Water

The Water organs are linked to our body's power and relate to life essence, the same essence that powers spiritual pursuit. Anyone who has spent time near an ocean, lake, or river can easily draw parallels to the movement of water and the currents of their own life. The wisdom of Water in Elemental Yin Yang Yoga however goes beyond the visible ebbs and flows you may have already noticed.

The Yin of Awareness and Intention

For yogis the concepts of awareness and intention are two we revisit regularly, but rarely connect one with the other. Several major changes have taken place in my life catalyzed by awareness practices and a reawakening of my purpose. One of the biggest shifts began when I added meditation to my daily routine. Although I had already been practicing and teaching yoga for years by that time, my main interest was in yang forms of yoga—fast-paced, physically demanding postures. I loved the feeling of having stress and stagnation washed from my body and mind after a challenging and energetic yoga class. At that time in my life I didn't fully appreciate the partnership between this style and slower yin forms of yoga.

When I finally committed to regular meditation, I found myself steeped in yin energy. For at least thirty minutes each day, I sat still without any mental or physical project to distract me. While seated meditation came with simple instructions, it was far more challenging than I had anticipated. Before long I realized that for years I had allowed my life to flow down a path I didn't like. Although I knew no one else was to blame for the mediocrity I was living in, I wasn't conscious of how I'd been shaping my current circumstances. In other words, I was not living a life I would have chosen for myself.

Once I became aware of how uncomfortable I was and how I wasn't working toward my dreams or living up to my own expectations, I couldn't ignore it. Within a few months of taking up meditation, I left a relationship, moved to a new home, took bold steps on my career path, and reduced my circle of friends to a few trusted and loved individuals. Regular awareness practice led me to a deeper understanding of myself and that is the mark of an effective tool.

At the beginning of the yoga journey, new awareness presents itself first in the body. Like a colour-blind person who can suddenly see various shades and hues they couldn't before, the yogi begins to experience sensations in the body more richly. Previously vague physical murmurs snap into focus and suddenly you can differentiate between pain and ease or tension and release more clearly. You may also notice greater mental and emotional awareness, which can assist you as you tease apart the internal jumble of your experiences. This clarity is an invitation to decide if what you are experiencing is how you want to feel and if you like the direction in which your life is moving. Awareness breeds intention when you allow your newfound clarity to penetrate your world on and off the mat.

The Yang of Will

Awareness for the sake of awareness isn't the end goal. The more in tune you become with your own currents and internal patterns, the more you will notice the consistencies and in-congruencies between your intentions and the reality of how you are living. Working with the Water element not only helps to you comprehend the deeper purpose and possible contributions you have to share with the world, but awareness can uncover the ways you may be unconsciously working against yourself. If you realize you are moving against your intended flow, it takes effort to redirect and form new patterns to support your goals. But in order to transform purpose into results, you need a strong will.

Sometimes this Water theme of will is thought of merely as willpower, but willpower without a strong intention is not enough to bring lasting change. For instance, think of a time in your life when you felt it might be time to transition to a more nutritious diet. Perhaps you saw a friend who quit sugar and looked incredible, or you read a study about how eating a certain way can improve your longevity. You make a sincere commitment to changing your lifestyle right then and there, but at dinner that night you realize you don't have any of the new foods you are "allowed" in your refrigerator and you go to bed with a grumbling belly. Within days you have exhausted your willpower trying desperately to resist the foods you want to eat in favour of the bland foods you've limited yourself to in your new program.

We have all experienced some version of this story, if not with food then with developing an exercise habit or when trying to cultivate a new practice or break an old, harmful pattern. The problem is often not with lack of willpower, but with a lack of a deep, specific personal intention and period of solid preparation to gather your resources.

I have seen people struggle for years to change their eating habits for vague or superficial reasons. Because they aren't clear on their ultimate goal they rarely take time to learn to cook healthier meals or use their resources to work with a knowledgeable nutritionist. The effort required usually ends up wasted in a cycle of guilt and failure. Interestingly, for some the real change begins when they land in the middle of a health crisis. Fear acts as a wake up call and suddenly their priorities become clear overnight. They drop their harmful habits and put their health needs first.

Willpower alone is not enough to sustain a long-term change for most people because it is a limited and draining energy. When your will is aligned with a deeply rooted purpose, however, and though it still takes energy to shift and grow, the desire to make a lasting change becomes a powerful ally that refuels you to help you move forward.

The Pursuit of Wisdom

"Fear is the emotion that arises in the face of the unknown. The sage through the clever utilization of resources and a focused will spends a lifetime cultivating wisdom. Wisdom is the virtue that empowers us to stand firmly in the face of the unknown and chart a steady course through uncertain waters."
~ **Lonny Jarrett**, *Nourishing Destiny*

As yogis and spiritual seekers we all hope to gain wisdom in our lives. Different than knowledge, which may be learned or passed along second-hand, wisdom is direct information that comes to you through lived experience. Wisdom has the power to change your perspective on life and on everything you thought you knew before.

For instance, if you want to learn about the experience of standing on the moon, you could read firsthand accounts about the steps it takes to become an astronaut and how the space shuttle moves through the various environments on its journey. You can spend time learning everything there is to know about the advanced science that makes it possible. But very few people have had that firsthand experience of standing on the moon and staring back at Earth. You can imagine into how it might feel, but only those who have been in that position after making that journey are in touch with the wisdom that those moments held for them. This may be a simplistic notion but I think of knowledge as something we learn from someone else and wisdom as something that unfolds through direct experience. Water relates to wisdom because wisdom is the antidote to fear, the emotion of water. Wisdom is the result of moving through the unknown even if fear is present.

Water: On the Mat

We have already explored several key themes of the Water element, but one that applies while on the yoga mat has to do with appropriate use of your energy and personal resources. Early in my yoga journey, I was involved with a vigorous and demanding asana practice called Ashtanga Yoga. Those who have achieved a level of mastery practicing this form of yoga have spent years turning it into a moving meditation and learning not to overexert or push beyond what is possible on any given day. I however, spent the first few years of my practice floundering. I would show up and go through the sequence with gusto only to exhaust myself and feel depleted for the rest of the day. Instead of returning to my mat the following morning I would convince myself that I had earned a "day off" which would turn into three days which would turn into a week. After that long break (long if you are aiming to have a daily practice), it would take a serious regrouping to gear up and get back on the mat.

This is not a unique story.

Perhaps you have a similar relationship with your yoga practice, your diet, your work, or your creative pursuits.

Working with the Water element is a way for us to learn, perhaps firstly on the mat, how to expend exactly the amount of energy necessary for the task at hand. In my classes I often see students making far too much effort to hold a posture, creating so much tension for the sake of "working hard" that I am concerned they may walk away from the mat with an injury, or just as damaging perhaps, with the wrong idea about yoga.

The wisdom of a Water practice is in learning how to use your resources intelligently. A simple way to work with this theme on your mat can be found in the exercise section at the end of this chapter.

Fear: The Emotion of Water

Fear is a primal and necessary human emotion. We are connected to fear so deeply that its alarm bells can stimulate the sympathetic nervous system (the fight or flight response) before you are conscious of feeling afraid. This part of your autonomic nervous system is a crucial, impersonal part of human survival. In moments of real or perceived danger, fear will fill you with the urge to fight or run away as your most basic instincts set in and your attention snaps to focus on the object of concern.

However useful this tool has been to the continuation of our species and our lives, fear can devastate our resources and qi. While the fear response is valuable if you are living in an environment that demands hyper vigilance, your brain can't tell the difference between a true threat and an imaginary disaster scenario you've drummed up from within. When fear is spent on things that have happened in your past or what you imagine could happen in the future, it will deplete your resources. If fear is a routine overreaction you have within a relatively safe and comfortable life, this hyperawareness can lead to exhaustion and paralyze you from doing anything outside your comfort zone or cause you to act recklessly instead of wisely.

On the other hand, fear can be a powerful motivator and catalyst for escaping dangerous situations. In the right moment, fear can kick start an impulse that saves your life or shakes you out of your status quo.

Water Constitution:
Nathan, the Ambitious Leader

Nathan is an important person in the sports industry. While not an athlete himself, he is manager to some of the nation's highest paid players. He is a shrewd negotiator who only accepts the very best contract deals and endorsements. While he can be difficult and demanding to work for, his staff learn more in a year working with Nathan than they would in a decade working for anyone else.

Nathan has a tight knit group of friends who adore him. He is brilliant, charismatic, and ambitious. These characteristics shine through and there is no shortage of people who want to date him. He exudes power and confidence and has a magnetic personality. Being seen with him can heighten someone's social status overnight whether they be a client or a love interest.

Behind closed doors however, life is not as wonderful. Nathan attends social and sports events nearly every night and because of it gets, on average, only four hours of sleep. He gives himself fully to every project he takes on and rarely allows himself downtime. Nathan can feel himself burning out, but since no one else has worked as hard to get on par with his superstar status it is difficult to lighten his load. Nathan has a hard time relinquishing control for fear of becoming obsolete in his industry. Although he has some strong friendships it is hard for him to form new relationships because so much of his energy is focused on work.

Those with Water constitutions easily find themselves in power positions because they tend to be determined and clear in their focus. However, when this element is excessive they may be power hungry and seem to only care about their goals and no one else's. Like a powerful wave or riptide sucking up everything around it, they can be overzealous and use their strength to get their way even if it leads to disastrous long-term results. Think of a CEO who ignores the feedback of the specialists on staff and ends up making an error that sets the company back several years and millions of dollars.

If someone is more of a deficient Water type, while they have desire to lead and others are drawn to them, they may not have the strength or skill to rally them once they are there. They feel easily defeated by their lack of resources and get worn down quickly.

Harmonized Water people on the other hand are incredible to be around. They exude drive and determination when they find purpose worthy of their energy. They champion important causes and mobilize others to dig deeper and find their purpose. A healthy Water individual flows easily around obstacles that appear in their path in order to move forward, and can make the most out of severely limited resources. Because Water types are so internally strong and confident, they don't feel threatened by others. Instead they use their resources to empower others in their field who may have a vision but lack the channels to see it through. A harmonized water individual can turn their lived experience into useful wisdom to share with the world and realize their life's purpose.

Water Exercise:
Using With Your Resources Wisely

Learning to work with your personal resources may sound simple but in reality it is a complicated endeavour. From an early age you may have learned to "give 100%" of your effort to every task put in front of you. Or perhaps you fear exhausting yourself and you work far below your capacity in order to avoid breaking a mental or physical sweat.

When it comes to energy output and using inner resources, the ideal would be to use exactly the amount of effort required to achieve your goals and move through life. When a task is simple you then wouldn't fuss over it, or feel obligated to give more than is needed. And when the time comes that you need to invest a large burst of energy to get you to the finish line, it would be available because you haven't depleted yourself using your resources frivolously.

One of the places you can start to investigate your own tendencies and use your personal resources wisely is on the yoga mat.

The 60% Practice

The next time you practice yoga, give it as much effort as you can. Do not push yourself to the point of injury, but do experience what it is like to give all you have. The practice following that, exert only 60% of your overall effort.

Notice the following:

- Which practice was more enjoyable?

- Which practice did you feel best after?

- Did the effort you exerted really change the depth and feel of the postures?

- What was your energy level like for the rest of the day after each practice?

Many people notice that the difference in the way they feel after each practice doesn't change much whether they extend more or less effort but their energy levels for the rest of the day following can be very different. Personally I find that I get the same benefit from my practice even working at 60% of my capacity but I don't feel drained or depleted the way I do after an exhausting workout or challenging practice.

Once you do this experiment you can start to refine how you use your personal resources on the mat. Look for signs from your body that you are pushing yourself beyond what is useful.

Some people experience:

- disconnection with the body and breath

- tension in an area of the body where it isn't required (i.e. the jaw, the brow, the shoulders)

- inner feelings of frustration or anxiety

- feelings of exhaustion

If you notice that much of your yoga practice is spent experiencing one or more of these things it may be time to reassess if you effort is being used wisely.

Once you have discovered how to notice and work with your inner re- sources on the mat, you can investigate and modify how you use your energy in all areas of your life.

Fire

"Beauty is not in the face; beauty is a light in the heart."
~ **Kahlil Gibran**

Hawaii

I stand with my feet buried in the soft sand. It is the end of February but the temperature is perfect. Last year at this time, I was in Boston watching a record breaking snowfall from my little apartment. I was newly pregnant, tired, and grumpy.

Such a contrast to this moment.

Standing beside my beloved husband with our beautiful baby in my arms, I stare out at the endless ocean. My feet immersed in the soft sand, I dip my daughter's toes into the warm water and she squeals as it rushes up the shoreline and quickly away again.

She won't remember this moment.

She won't remember the adventure we have had together over the last month travelling around the islands, hiking on the side of a dormant volcano, playing in the sand, and watching surfers ride the waves. She won't remember any of it, but I will never forget what this time has meant to me.

Somewhere down the beach we hear the sound of a conch and the Hawaiian prayer to the setting sun is called. The baby coos along with the chant and together we watch the sun make its descent into the ocean,

Fire returning to Water. Yang returning to yin. I stand here basking in the embrace of my little family and feel my heart swell with devotion and profound love.

I remember when I was younger, love felt so complicated. My relationships were often wracked with tension, discord, miscommunication and misunderstanding.

My husband kisses my forehead and my awareness rushes back gratefully to the present. I finally understand that love can be simple and warm and free of pain and drama.

We stand together with our daughter as the sky grows darker, enjoying the perfection and warmth of this moment.

Fire

The Element of Fire is given an honoured place in many traditions. It is a universal symbol for life, love, and the sun. Learning to build and harness fire as a tool is one of the pivotal moments in early human history allowing our ancient ancestors the ability to stay warm, cook food, and engage in life after dark. In Chinese philosophy, Fire holds the position as divine Emperor or Empress. While Water is the most yin of the elements, Fire is the most yang. It is a warm embrace, the beating heart, the gift of summer and sunlight, a powerful protector and destroyer.

The Season of Fire: Summer

Nearly every living thing on this planet depends on the sun's energy for life and, in areas of the world that experience four distinct seasons, summer is the traditional time of the summer solstice. After the long winter and fluctuating temperatures of spring, it is finally time to enjoy long, lazy days frolicking outdoors. Summer is a time for celebration, popular for weddings and vacations as the hours of yang-fuelled warmth and sunlight, and the season itself, offer the perfect backdrop to to revel in the beauty and abundance of life.

Summer is the most yang season, because it is the warmest and brightest. For the yogi, summer is a satisfying point along the wheel of the year to play on the mat. Since it takes less time and effort to get physically warmed up, summer allows you to focus more creatively on exploring and expanding your practice in ways you might not be open to during the rest of the year.

The Organs

Fire is a special element not only because of its role as monarch, the Emperor or Empress of the Five Element system, but also because Fire rules not just one yin and one yang organ but two of each.

The Fire Yin Organs

The yin organs for each element are tasked with the important job of storing a person's life-force energy, or qi, and blood. These organs are integral to life because they deal directly with the both the essences needed to live and our most important physiological functions. While you can live without your gallbladder (a yang organ), you cannot live without your heart (a yin Fire organ). This is why the yin organs are so revered in the Chinese Medicine system and must be protected and nurtured.

The Heart - The Emperor or Empress

Just as the sun is of central importance to life on Earth, the Heart is essential for each individual's life. The heart begins to beat long before birth and when it finally rests, life ceases to be. It is a constant companion in nearly every animal's life, working tirelessly to move blood to every cell within the body.

It is no wonder in Chinese Philosophy that the Heart has earned the highest honour, the role of the Emperor or Empress. While our connection with an all powerful, divinely ordained monarchy may not be culturally relevant today, the Heart is like an Emperor from a beautiful fairytale. Groomed for his position from birth, the sole purpose of his life is to consider and care for the entire nation, every day and without fail.

If however the ruler is corrupt, he will only allocate resources to his friends and to areas of the Empire that he has a vested interested in. In the body, this kind of dysfunction will eventually prove disastrous: certain areas of the body can be flooded with blood that isn't needed while others are undernourished, requiring other organs to work harder to deal with a lack of blood supply.

No other person in the Empire has the birthright to perform the job of the Emperor just as no other organ can do the job of the Heart. That is why it is important to cultivate healthy Fire energy. The healthy Emperor or Empress understands the importance of every person, from her most valued counsellor to the farmer who lives on the country's borderlands; similarly, the healthy heart pumps nutrients all over the body and must insure that lifeblood reaches every corner of the domain within its care.

The Pericardium - The Emperor's Personal Guard

If the Heart is the Emperor, then the Pericardium is his personal body-guard. In the anatomical body, the Pericardium is not an organ at all, but a membrane around the Heart protecting it from illness and devastating emotional fluctuations. Without its bodyguard, the Heart would be like a house with no walls, subject to the onslaught of the ever-changing weather.

A healthy Pericardium not only prevents strong emotions or illness from damaging the Heart, but it acts as a two-way filter. Like a devoted companion, the Pericardium uses protective discretion in deciding who and what gets an audience with the Emperor and how things are communicated back out into the world.

The Fire Yang Organs

The yang organs differ in function from their yin counterparts. While the yin organs store and interact with the vital substances of the body, the yang organs are more like portals constantly being filled and emptied. The yang organs do not deal with the vital substances directly but instead work with food and waste products. They are important, however, in fuelling the body and providing the raw materials for qi and blood.

The Small Intestine - The Receptionist/ Alchemist

In one of the famous Chinese Medicine texts, The Yellow Emperor's Classic, the Small Intestine is known as the Reception official. A good receptionist greets a visitor and quickly determines first if they get past the front door into the court of the Emperor. The Emperor has a very important job and, therefore, more often than not, the Receptionist takes a message, boils it down to its most basic essentials and passes it along.

In Western medicine, the role of the small intestine is similar. It is in charge of absorbing the majority of nutrients from the food and passing along the leftovers to be further sorted or turned into waste and eliminated further down the gastrointestinal tract. In Elemental Yin Yang theory the Small Intestine is also an Alchemist, filtering and distilling down the ingredients that come into the body until she is left with "gold" the amino acids and some of the nutrients needed to keep the Heart and the rest of the body healthy. The Small Intestine is involved with clarity of mind and discernment since it must decide what is relevant to share with the Heart in order for it to get the pure essence of the message.

The Triple Burner - The Irrigation Official

While not an organ of the physical body, the Triple Burner is known in The Yellow Emperor's Classic as the Irrigation official. It may not be a glamorous job, but it is an important one. Without a solid irrigation system on a farm, crops would be fed unevenly and flooding would be inevitable in one area while another thirsted for water. In the same way that you don't notice the sewage system in your city until there is a problem, this official is often operating under the radar.

Besides of its duties for the transportation of water and waste, the Triple Burner is also said to be a motivator for all physiological functions (yang activities) of the body. If one of the organs is not working correctly or starts hoarding resources—creating a supply crisis for everyone else down the line—the situation can quickly become hostile and urgent. The Triple Burner has the job of stepping in to offer mediation, a pep talk, or even to redirect resources in order to solve the issue and bring the system back to a harmonious, cooperative place.

Themes of Fire

Love and Connection

Fire deals with all forms of love. From the passion found in a kiss to the moment a parent hears the cry of their baby for the first time. Beyond the warm feelings and deep care we feel for that which we cherish, love—at its core—is about connection. In fact, the word yoga means "to yoke." Union is the essential teaching of the Fire element not only because of its importance as a spiritual realization but because it is a fundamental pillar of our existence.

Spend enough time in spiritual circles and you will hear the sentiment "we are all One," even though most people don't feel that way in their day-to-day lives. Interestingly, this is also the reason many set out on the yogic path. They are searching for a felt sense of deep connection. Ironically, whether you feel it or not, you are swimming in connection. You literally could not live without it.

At birth, you are one of the most vulnerable mammals on the planet. Some newborn animals, unlike human babies, can walk and run within hours of coming into the world. The survival of you as a newborn child depends on the deep connection between you and your primary care-givers. You also depend on innovations of humans who came before you. The development of medicine, architecture, agriculture, and count-less other developments have shaped culture and provided ways for our species not only to survive but to thrive.

Our connection to the world around us is even more rudimentary when you consider that the human body relies on a very specific exterior envi-ronment. If the earth's temperature, gravitational field, or ratio of oxygen to carbon dioxide were to change even slightly the planet would be un-inhabitable for human life. From this perspective, human life is actually quite vulnerable and depends on a holistic connection with the people and the environment we live in.

And yet, despite all the ways we are connected to and a part of our world many still live with the false belief that they are isolated and alone. The most important teaching of the Fire element is that we are swimming in love and connection even when we don't feel the spark. Working closely with this element is a reminder that every beat of your heart will help keep the lines open between you and the world as a whole.

Mature Love

Imagine you are in a new relationship with someone. Things are going well, you are in love, and then suddenly they start waking you up at three o'clock in the morning every night screaming,

"Make me a sandwich!"

You run to the kitchen and make them some food. When you get back they are sitting up in the bed with wide eyes laughing hysterically.

"I wet the bed. Give me a bath and clean me up."

Thirty minutes later you have your beloved all cleaned up and fed but now they won't go back to sleep. "Can you carry me around the house for a while?" They whine.

You know it is a ridiculous request but when you hesitate they start screaming again, so you gather them up in your arms. For several hours you carry them until they finally fall asleep. With burning arms and an aching back you set them down and tuck yourself back in to bed exhausted. Soon after, your alarm goes off and it is time to get ready for work.

If you were in a relationship and your partner started making these ridiculous demands my guess is that your warm feelings would evaporate in a heartbeat. Many parents, however, play out some version of this scenario on a nightly basis with their children. The kind of love one feels for a child is different from the love you feel for a partner. The first, based on deep biological programming, feels more like blind devotion. The love for a partner, in contrast, deals with the Fire theme of maturity. While all forms of love are within Fire's domain, mature love based in reciprocity and respect is one of the key teachings of this element. Romantic love may begin because of mutual attraction, but it typically won't grow and evolve into a long-term, fulfilling, mature partnership in the absence of shared values, and without respect as well as the enjoyment of the other that brought you together in the beginning.

There is no denying that new love feels wonderful at first, and there is absolutely nothing wrong with that. But if the flames of that love are stoked by fantasies, assumptions about who the other person is, and what life with them will be like, it can blind you—to such a degree that it is easy to miss the reality of who the other person truly is. This may lead to the path of heartbreak and disillusionment later on.

Mature love on the other hand may not feel giddy and thrilling in the same way a new relationship is, but it is rooted in trust and care that has been communicated and cultivated over time. This love is sacred to Fire and takes courage to engage in since you are letting another into your Heart. Mature love allows you to share not only the polished version of yourself that you project out into the world, but also the most vulnerable and fragile parts of who you are.

Fire: On the Mat

For the Elemental yogi, Fire practice is one of connection. Yoga, as I've mentioned, means to "yoke" after all. Recognizing the union with the entire universe we are part of is one of the most simple yet profound spiritual mysteries. On the mat, asana practice is the opportunity to remember that we are connected to our universe and each other in ways both basic and profound.

In my Fire yoga classes, for the last yang posture (usually the most vigorous and challenging of the practice) I ask my students to get into groups. In those groups the student must rely on their partners for support in the posture.

At first it may be awkward.

Most people are accustomed to practicing yoga in a class with others, but it is rare to step out of the boundary of your own mat, meet another student, and together work towards new insight and understanding in a posture. Suddenly you may be practicing a physically challenging pose and relying on a total stranger to support you. In a supported handstand you may come face to face with your own vulnerability or boundaries around trust.

For the Fire element, this intimate sharing of the practice can be a huge challenge. You may dislike having to break out of your own flow to get into a relationship with the person practicing beside you. You might also find that working with another student brings needed inspiration to your practice. They see something you didn't notice or encourage you away from the belief that you "can't" do a particular pose before you give it a try.

These moments in class are what I live for as a teacher. Seeing someone believe they aren't strong enough or "good" enough to attempt a pose and then witness a group of peers playfully inspire them to give it a try by promising them support and a cheering section is a beautiful thing. Whether the person "gets" the pose or not isn't important. The mutual love of the practice, along with kindness and connection between yogis, is the real heart of the moment. At that apex of the class session, the room bubbles over with laughter and, very often, the same person who claimed that handstand was impossible for them has surprised themselves as they smile at their team while happily hanging upside down.

This begs the question, if you can achieve the "impossible" on your mat by simply and playfully giving it a shot, what have you been shying away from in your life that may also be within your grasp?

Boundaries

For yogis the flip side of believing that you aren't strong enough or experienced enough for a certain posture is pushing yourself in the name of asana glory. Since the Fire element deals with boundaries through the Pericardium, or Emperor's guard, working with this element is especially important for A-type students who are driven not only on the mat, but in all aspects of life.

The Fire postures include a collection of "heart openers." Typically backbends, these asanas require not only supple shoulders, hips, thighs, and a healthy spine, but also a tremendous amount of strength. If you push a backbend too far using brute strength to muscle your way beyond the flexibility you lack, it could result in serious injury. Likewise if you are hypermobile, without the stability needed to safely navigate a backbend, you open yourself up to an injury in the spine or shoulders.

Healthy Fire energy in a yogi is exhibited by being open to deeper possibilities for themselves while still respecting that "openings"—mental, physical, and even spiritual—may take time.

Unfortunately, many yoga practitioners become addicted to their practice and yearn for deeper, ever intensifying sensations of stretch or the glory of a more aesthetically beautiful practice. In the yoga world, the phenomenon of gymnasts and ex-dancers posing for beautiful pictures in advanced asana has driven many a well-meaning yogi to believe that one must bend themselves into elaborate shapes (that have little value for the average body who only practices a few times a week, if that) in order to be considered an accomplished yoga practitioner.

Working with Fire energy on the mat can allow you to stay connected, not only with greater possibilities for yourself but in order to maintain healthy and mature boundaries concerning what is realistic for you during your practice on any given day. At the same time, Fire energy allows you to enjoy what your body is able to do without comparing yourself to those images of a gymnast turned yogi.

Joy: The Emotion of Fire

When viewing life from the Five Element system of the emotions, the emotion ruled by Fire certainly stands out. Unlike the other four emotions—grief (Metal), worry (Earth), anger (Wood), and fear (Water), joy seems like a positive force compared to its companions. While the emotion of joy is one we would choose over all the others if given the choice, there is another side to feelings of overwhelming pleasure.

Joy is beautiful. How could it ever be harmful?

As previously mentioned, if you have ever fallen in love (or lust) you know how exhilarating a feeling it can be. You feel alive and awake, and the whole world seems to shimmer a little bit more. Someone newly in love or "love sick," finds that they can't eat or sleep, or concentrate on anything but the object of their desire.

If the new relationship lasts and the "high" continues, the lovebirds may neglect all other relationships in their life in order to spend every waking moment with their beloved. They may be so engrossed they put themselves in harm's way and fail to pay attention to the stop sign in front of them (both literally and metaphorically).

In this way, unmitigated joy, or what we think of as joy, can be more like a type of mania. The once grounded, rational individual begins to play the part of an addict looking for more fuel to feed their burning passion.

The Fire theme of maturity plays an important role here and, for most people, the fires of extreme joy will be tamed, contained, and transformed into useful energy and a more subtle, sustainable, and pleasant happiness. Healthy joy is the type that is allowed to pass through you. It feels wonderful, especially compared to the other emotions. Like the other four emotions, it is a natural response to life and only becomes problematic if you try to cling to it or chase it.

Fire Constitution:
Ashley, The Local Celebrity

When Ashley walks into a room, she lights it up with her smile. It isn't hard to see why people love her. She is articulate and funny, and when she is paying attention to you, you feel connected and part of the "in-crowd." Ashley conveys such personal warmth that even strangers feel immediately comfortable and at ease, like old friends, in her company. It isn't hard to see why people love her. She has passionate (although short-lived) relationships and wherever you go with her you feel that you are part of the entourage of a huge celebrity. Stereotypical as it may be, she is like the sun and everyone orbits around her.

However, Ashley has a hard time saying no. Because people love to be around her and she makes everyone feel like her best friend, people feel that they have a claim on her. Ironically it is often difficult to connect with Ashley on a deep level because someone else is always in line vying for her attention. Her close friends often complain that they need to schedule one-on-one time with her months in advance and then inevitably she is double booked and brings other people along for the ride. The people close to her can easily feel jealous because she isn't available for them as much as they would hope.

Although she admits she spreads herself too thin and feels anxious about how much she is juggling, she detests being alone or without a packed calendar to make her feel important and busy. Outwardly, Ashley seems to have the world at her fingertips, but she often feels trapped by the increasing demands of her relationships, burning out quickly. She turns to stimulants and love affairs to boost her energy and her mood so she can fulfill the demands on her time that she has shackled herself to.

A Fire type or someone with Fire disharmony, may find themselves hungry for joy the way a storm chaser is for a storm. Fire constitutions have a strong tendency to pursue highs and thrills in all aspects of their lives: their work, their relationships, and their physical practices. They may find themselves getting bored once anything becomes routine. This can help Fire individuals be innovative and open to new and creative ways of doing things. But when Fire energy is excessive they may jump from thing to thing, relationship to relationship, burning bridges and burning out.

In contrast, one who lacks sufficient fire may seem cold and lifeless in their dealings. They may recoil from any felt connection or be hypervigilant about their emotional boundaries.

A harmonized Fire person can be intoxicating to be around. Other constitutions flock to their warmth and kindness and their offer of love and inclusion. These individuals are connected to what their larger purpose in life is. Like the Emperor that rules the nation, the harmonized Fire type can communicate well, hold appropriate boundaries with the various and complex relationships they have, and easily command the attention of those around them.

Fire Exercise: A Morning Ritual

Spiritual life enchanted me over twenty years ago. When I was a young teenager I started to dabble in yoga, tarot cards and mystical teachings of various spiritual schools and religions. While my primary path followed celebrating seasons and moon cycles, all forms and expressions of harmonious living with both the natural world and one another intrigued me.

Even with the conscious effort to keep a felt sense of connection to the world around me, it was difficult. At points in my life I lived in the middle of a big city with no access to hiking trails. Other times I lived far away from family and friends and didn't feel the joyful connection that one gets in the presence of those who know and love you.

However, there was one consistent practice that I adopted in my early days as a spiritual seeker that helped me acknowledge the reality that we are always connected to our world and to one another even when we don't feel it in our experience.

Call it prayer, or an active meditation but this morning ritual was a companion to me for much of the last two decades to help ignite the themes of the Fire Element. I provide this morning ritual to you as an example. You may wish to do this before your morning yoga or meditation practice, but do adapt it to suit you own style and religious or spiritual beliefs. The most powerful prayer or ritual is the one you craft for yourself. from your own heart.

Awakening Fire

When you wake up, find a quiet spot in your living space. If you wish, light a candle or sit near a window that allows the morning light in (if you are an early riser do this short ritual at sunrise).

Sit in silence for a moment.

Turn your attention to your heartbeat. Notice its rhythm and marvel in its dutiful service in your life.

Acknowledge a few of the ways that you are connected to others deeply even sitting still right now. For instance, if you are siting on a cushion, how many people did it take to produce the various materials within it, put them together, send them to the shop you got it from?
How many people made it possible for that store to exist?
If you are sitting in a house with electricity, how many people are integral to that process?

Allow yourself to be overwhelmed by how many people and different systems you depend on just to be sitting here quiet and comfortable.

Next think of the different ways your presence in the world influences others. How many people are potentially affected by your work?
If you support others how does your care trickle out to into the world?

Bring your attention back to your heartbeat and say the following prayer or craft one of your own.

"Beautiful Heart, Inner Emperor/ Empress
I bow to You who holds my deepest purpose and vision.
May your light penetrate all that I am and all that I do.
Thank you for your service to my body, mind and soul as I
strive to live a connected and conscious life.
Full of love, Namaste/Amen/Blessed Be."

If you are continuing with a yoga or meditation practice do so; when you are finished snuff out the candle and move into the next phase of your day.

Wood

"They [the spirits of wood] endow us with the ability to discern our path, stay clear on our direction, imagine possibilities, move forward toward our goals and take a stand for what we believe is right."
~**Lorie Dechar**, *Five Spirits: Alchemical Acupuncture for Psychological and Spiritual Healing*

Perspective and the Path

For a morning in early April, it is warm. Although the weather has oscillated back and forth from chilly to mild in the last few days, today it feels like spring is finally breaking through.

I step out on the trail. It is muddy and there are clumps of ice still hiding in shadows that the sun can't reach, but the smell of spring is unmistakable. The promise of warmer days kisses my face in the soft breeze. As I walk deeper into the forest, I notice little buds beginning to burst in every direction.

In a matter of weeks the forest will be lush and green once again, but at this moment it is on the verge of transformation, filled with possibility. No matter how many times I walk this path, I never cease to be captivated by the beauty here. I start to climb the hill and notice that my mood has lifted and the concerns that brought me here have faded temporarily into the background.

I am at a crossroads in my life, unsure of where to focus my energy, unable to choose a direction for fear of "missing out" on other opportunities. Somehow being surrounded by the rapid growth happening naturally here in the forest is soothing.

Not only is the surrounding environment beautiful, it provides me with a different perspective on how to move forward in life. The trees don't wait for someone to validate their yearning towards majestic height, they just grow. The flowers don't hide because they might not be ready, they simply bloom.

And yet, life offers no guarantees. A tree might be blown over in a storm, the flower plucked from the ground at the peak of its beauty. That doesn't stop them from relentlessly expressing their true nature and following their path.

Without giving me advice, the Wood element has offered me its wisdom here today. Vision and potential are only meaningful if you use them. While we can never know exactly where our path may lead, it would be a tragedy to live out our lives standing at a fork in the road unable to decide which way to go.

Wood

Wood may be unfamiliar to those newer to the exploration of Five Elements, however, the themes and symbols of this element make Wood quickly useful and accessible to the Elemental Yin Yang yogi. The magic of this element can both inspire and empower you to reach for your big dreams and forge the life you truly want to live.

The Season of Wood: Spring

Spring is a time of rebirth, renewal, and, above all, possibility. There is a magical quality to the air. It smells fresh and sweet as the earth shakes off its snowy coat and tiny plants begin to reach up towards the sun.

Before technological advances that have allowed much of the world to enjoy heated homes and buildings to do our work, spring was a time of celebration. It was the turning point in the year when the community knew they had survived the harsh winter and life would go on. In nature, spring is a popular time for animals to begin the dance of procreation. Their resources have lasted them through the winter and they are ready to mate again.

In our lives, spring is the metaphor for youth. It is the time when there is more potential than concrete direction. It is miraculous that a tiny sprout can grow into a majestic tree just as a newborn will develop into a fully grown, independent adult. The potential held here is a yearly reminder that if the conditions are right, growth can and will occur both in nature and within ourselves.

The Organs

Wood Yin: The Liver - The General

In the elemental fairytale, the yin organ for Wood may not strike you as overly yin in nature. The Liver holds the role of general in the army of the Empress. As a military leader, this organ is in charge of strategy for offensive protection. An overly ambitious general may push his troops too far or sacrifice them without cause in order to chase glory. However, an organized and rational military leader knows how to inspire the respect of his soldiers, unite them against their enemies, and under no circumstance ever minimizes the role they play in the protection of the Empire. He also has done the work to gain self-knowledge—he has a clear inner perspective and is aware of his personal strengths and weaknesses, of how his personality will play into the dynamics of the leadership of the country. No energy is wasted because everyone knows their role. The path has been set and the goal is clear.

In the Chinese Medicine model of the body, the Liver is a yin organ because it acts as a container for blood and orchestrates the smooth movement of qi in the body. When blood is plentiful and qi is moving the way it should, the Liver is content, but if there is a weak link in the chain, the Liver can become an irritable and angry general. Many women experience this on a monthly basis as they prepare for menstruation. Until the qi and blood begin to move, it is common to experience some premenstrual irritability.

Wood Yang: The Gall Bladder - The Judge

Unlike the other yang organs that deal directly with food, water, and waste, the Gall Bladder deals with bile. Its main function is to store and release bile as needed for the digestion process. The Gall Bladder also is considered the highest ranking judge in the Empire. This official is in charge of making decisions, weighing pros and cons with the impact of taking one direction over another. A disempowered judge may have a hard time owning their role in the courtroom and trouble coming to a decision. A strong judge, however, will express the qualities of being courageous and decisive, and will provide the tools to follow through on the appointed path.

Wood Themes

When understood, the characteristics of this element can offer philosophical and practical assistance in the realization your life's goals and aspirations. Not only that, but they are incredible instructions for meditation if that practice is a companion on your life journey.

To understand the three core characteristics of the Wood element we'll use the metaphor of a tree.

The Roots: Grounding and Foundation

When standing in the presence of a breathtaking tree, it is easy to forget that what you are looking at is only part of the picture. Beneath the earth is a system of roots that spread deep and wide, gathering nutrients and forming the foundation of the tree. Without the roots, the tree wouldn't have access to the energy it needs to flourish nor would it be grounded enough to withstand a periodic pummelling by a strong wind.

In our lives it is much the same. You can't earn a degree or build a business overnight. It takes years of study, long hours, and the commitment to overcome obstacles. There may be no one to witness and appreciate your hard work as you strengthen your foundation for the future. In fact, the more intense the goal, the deeper the roots need to be. Long-term growth and success is rarely possible without a strong foundation, which often won't receive any accolades along the way. And yet, just as we may forget about that intricate root system beneath the forest floor, it is easy to forget the years of "behind the scenes" work that went into someone's success when viewed from the outside.

The roots of a tree are a metaphor for commitment to a path or goal and taking a stand in order to achieve something further down the road. Through practices like yoga or meditation you consciously work to ground yourself and set a foundation of perspective and clarity for your daily life. This is one aspect of the Wood element in action. It teaches us that in order to know who you are and to realize your life purpose you must make the time and space to develop your foundation. In order to complete a marathon, an intelligent person will spend months training. It would be unwise to attempt such a huge physical and mental feat the first day you decided to give running a try.

The Trunk: Focus

While the roots are the unsung heroes of the tree structure, the trunk is the strong single-pointed part of the tree that supports the height and weight of the upper leaves and branches. It carries nutrients back and forth and is always in conversation with your foundation (roots) and aspiration (crown). The trunk is a metaphor for focus and determination to reach your highest goals.

While the roots and leaves spread to absorb as much as possible, the trunk stays focused and specific in its work. A thriving tree has a central body that allows the crown of leaves and branches to spread far and wide. The energy of the trunk is a metaphor for the health of the Wood element within you. It represents the fortitude to put your head down and do the work it will take to move forward and stay firm in your personal commitment.

Focus however is not simply about staying on task, it is also the ability to discern what to let into your field and when to say no to things that aren't going to help you grow or realize your goal. For example, when writing this book I had to decline numerous social invitations and short-term-gain career opportunities because they didn't align with my vision and timeline for completing this project.

Another important teaching from the Wood element when working with a big dream is to form a clear structure and break down the path into tangible steps while avoiding what I call "Big-Dream Paralysis." Perhaps you have a moment when a brilliant, ambitious goal strikes you, and you feel ecstatic, inspired, and excited. You tell a few trusted friends about your new idea and begin plotting your next move.

Not long after, you hit a wall.

You realize that in order to jump-start your big dream you will need funds you don't have, more education, and a huge shift in lifestyle. Suddenly the way forward becomes unclear and you don't know how to turn your dream into reality. Doubt creeps in and, like a slow moving poison, it contaminates the purity of your idea bit by bit until you force yourself to stop thinking about it all together. It's too big, too overwhelming.

This has probably happened to you several times in your life. Overwhelmed by the magnitude of a big dream, you squashed the whole thing entirely because there wasn't a clear path.

The Wood element is not only concerned with perspective and the ability to dream your dreams but can also help you break those goals down into actionable, reasonable steps that will get you there. The trunk of the tree represents the diligence, hard work, and unification of mind, body, and soul that is often required to realize our wildest and most important aspirations.

The Crown: Freedom and Letting Go

While the roots stay firm and the trunk bends only slightly, the crown of the tree is free to dance in the wind and bask in the light of inspiration and new perspectives without fear. The upward spreading of branches and leaves represent perspective and freedom as a result of strong foundation and focused determination.

The crown is also the part that symbolizes letting go with grace. In the autumn, trees shed their leaves in order to conserve energy and survive winter. In your own life knowing how to let go with grace is an art. Perhaps you set out to achieve a specific goal and after reaching a plateau found that the view was not what you expected. You didn't like the direction you were heading. Or you realized you didn't have the resources to continue to grow into your plan. From this view point, with a bigger perspective than when you began, you have the option to be flexible and shift your course with grace and clarify what is needed next. New information and an attitude of openness allow you to pivot as needed rather than adhere stubbornly to a course that no longer supports your evolving goals.

Wood: On the Mat

The Wood element has an abundance of wisdom to share both on and off the mat. An Elemental Yin Yang Yoga practice specifically geared to the Wood element is a perfect opportunity to work on physical stamina or approach postures you would like to move more deeply into. Wood, being upright and goal and growth oriented, invites you to expand beyond what you believe to be possible for yourself and shake up the status quo.

In the Elemental Yin Yang classes I teach, one way I access Wood yang energy is through a vigorous yet playful bootcamp style of postures and pacing. I offer my students asanas that are challenging, strengthening, and may require just an ounce more energy than they normally exert (but not so much that they leave class feeling depleted). Since Wood is in charge of the smooth flow of qi, a vigorous flow helps flush the body of stagnation and clear the path for qi and blood to move optimally.

In a Wood yin practice, my approach focuses more on this element's emotion. I once heard a teacher say that the pose doesn't begin until the student feels uncomfortable. I don't interpret this to mean physically uncomfortable or potentially injurious, but instead when the student wants to get out of the posture for other reasons.

For example when a long-held pose becomes mentally uncomfortable you may experience boredom or irritation. In any other situation, when you aren't enjoying the experience you likely remove yourself fairly quickly or search for a distraction. Most of us check our phones incessantly to avoid the boredom of waiting for a bus or cross the street to avoid having to talk to our long-winded neighbour. However in a yin yoga pose, our boredom or slight irritability is a perfect moment to sit a little longer and either observe how you deal with unpleasant feelings.

The point is not to learn how to put up with negative situations, sensations or people, the point is to find tools besides distraction, avoidance or anger when you do have to deal with occasional and inevitable discomfort in your life. For those who want a deeper challenge in the yin practice when the urge to move out of the pose arises, rather than exploring your tools to manage your response, you can simply let the boredom or irritation be exactly as it is.

The Wood element, like some of the other elements, teaches you how to use your time on the mat to stay inspired without getting stuck on your self-imposed mental blockages. It also gives you the space to allow your honest experiences to come up without having to cure, fix, or hide the things you don't enjoy. Working with the Wood element is to walk a path toward greater perspective in order to see things the way they are— the best elixir for feeling clear and motivated to live out your dreams.

Anger: The Emotion of Wood

Of all the emotions in Chinese Medicine anger may be the most difficult to resolve for yogis, or anyone for that matter. As you engage in spiritual life no doubt you have been taught that anger is "unyogic" and divisive. It is easy to see that most other emotions have the power to unite people. We commiserate and console in times of grief, laugh together in moments of joy, and reach out for comfort and support in our fear or worry.

Anger however is typically seen as an exclusively dangerous, untamable emotion that "spiritual" people must cure or transcend. During moments of true anger, it is difficult to keep a larger perspective and conduct yourself with dignity and integrity (some of the more positive sign posts of healthy Wood). If anger is chronic, mismanaged, or suppressed it can rot someone from the inside out, twisting their mind and heart until they have forgotten the greater purpose of their life. A burst of violent anger can instantly ruin lives through words and actions. It is not surprising that we find it difficult to see redeeming qualities in this emotion.

When used creatively and intelligently, however, there are positive uses for this force. While it cannot be sustained for too long, anger can gift us with motivation, it can rally an individual's resources to leave a dysfunctional relationship, or walk away from a job that is slowly corroding their soul. Bubbling anger over injustice in the world is the root of all revolutions and often the energetic catalyst needed to set plans into motion that prompt fundamental shifts. Time and time again major cultural movements erupt when enough people get fed up with class division, racism, sexism, and other social or environmental issues. Anger is not enough to bring about lasting change, but it can be a powerful tool that unites the focused effort of an individual or group toward a specific goal. While it cannot be sustained for long, if anger isn't expressed in a healthy and constructive way it can simmer for years and poison new growth.

The Importance of Anger

Anger is generally difficult and uncomfortable, but that doesn't mean it doesn't have a role to play. If you have been taught that your anger isn't allowed or that you are a childish or reactive for feeling it, I encourage you, all of us really, to look at it from a different perspective.

Consider physical pain. Everyone knows that physical pain feels bad, and yet it is one way our body keeps us safe and calls us to pay attention to it when something is awry. Much like anger, pain is highly unpleasant and yet one of the most dangerous conditions someone can have is a congenital insensitivity to this physical alarm.

From a young age, children are taught to avoid things that result in pain, and that conditioned response is key to our survival. You can tell a young child a dozen times not to touch a hot pan because it is danger-ous. However when that mischievous little person does it anyway, the resulting experience of pain is the final and firm message they receive to never do it again.

Pain is a harsh teacher but a teacher nonetheless. Through it one learns not to do things that are dangerous or harmful.

Anger is very similar. It is an alert from within that something is wrong. If you constantly suppress anger and don't make the space to investigate its source, you could end up much like someone that can't feel physical pain. Gloss over the important signals that something is wrong or unjust and over time you may end up with no personal power and in a dangerous situation—physically and/or emotionally.

While it is true that any expression of anger has consequences, the Elemental yogi can direct that expression consciously to fuel creative projects or kickstart a new path.

At the end of this chapter, I've provided suggestions for harnessing this volatile emotion in a creative and productive way.

Wood Constitution:
Bill, The Entrepreneur

Bill is a focused guy. In the past ten years he has started two different businesses that both continue to enjoy success. When people ask him his secret to success and staying motivated, he insists that it all comes down to meticulous planning and the stubbornness to continue regardless of setbacks.

A new father of twins, Bill has had to learn to be a bit more flexible when it comes to work in order to deal with ever-changing routines as a parent. Although he tries to adhere to all the deadlines and goals he has set for himself, the two little people in his life often have other plans. One may be up all night crying while the other comes down with a cold the next day. Bill loves his children deeply and hopes that as they grow they will inherit his initiative and strive toward their big dreams as well.

Bill is full of life and energy and some people find his booming voice and personality intimidating. Although he is generally even tempered he has been known to get into heated arguments over small, unimportant details and those closest to him know that when he is in a bad mood it is best to leave him alone. Bill doesn't enjoy the part of himself that struggles with dissatisfaction and anger, but when it rains it pours, and he can't escape the feeling that the bad days are out to get him.

Those who are primarily Wood tend to have their eye on the prize. This is not to say that all goal-oriented people are Wood types, because any constitution will have their own brand of focus and technique for personal development, but someone who is Wood will likely set a goal and stick to the plan no matter which way the wind blows.

Wood people have a special relationship with ambitious goals and plans. Those who a lack sufficient dose of this energy may be easily confused when they set out to dream big and have trouble following through. Those who have excessive Wood energy may plough forward even when they get information that should change their initial mapped course. These types hate to deviate in any way from their plan because once they make the decision to do something, any detour, for them, feels like failure.

Quitting is not something Wood types take kindly to. They may finish something for the sake of finishing it even if the process has gone cold or is clearly fruitless. In fact, many with this excessive pattern will both ignore clear signs along the path and then feel anger when they don't get the results they wanted, and may even feel victimized.

Healthy Wood energy, whether it is an individual's primary constitution or simply in the mix with the other elements, is the ability to hold a wide perspective and see different possibilities while simultaneously moving toward goals and commitments. They can harness their passion and take the steps towards change and growth. Historically, many powerful activists were Wood constitutions, who not only spoke out against injustice but, spearheaded by their dissatisfaction, organized movements to shake culture out of the status quo.

Wood Exercise: Working With Anger

While Anger may not feel good, it is an alarm from within that deserves your attention. Here are a few ways to work with anger and learn to use it or diffuse it.

1. Acknowledge

The next time anger starts to bubble up instead of demonizing it, suppressing it or avoiding it altogether, simply acknowledge what you are feeling. Conversely if your tendency is to let anger overrule your better judgment, name the physical or emotional qualities.

"I feel my face getting hot and a tension in my abdomen".

2. Make Space

Much like a mindfulness meditation, the act of observing and naming what is happening in your awareness trains you to have more space between your present experience and your reaction to it.

That space is power.

An extra few seconds of observation is often enough to give you the time to re-think whatever words are about to come flying out of your mouth and abate any destructive or thoughtless action. That space will also give you the opportunity to step away from the source of your anger for a moment, gracing you with more time to take the next step with a deeper awareness of future consequences.

3. Seek Wider Perspective

The antidote to anger is often perspective. While there may be countless examples of wrongdoing in the world, the truth of most conflicts is often nuanced. In your own life you have no doubt been the focus of someone's anger because the other person did not have all of the details of the situation. Perhaps as a child your sibling got angry at you for taking a toy out of their room without asking. They yell at you and run crying to your mother that you "stole" their toy. Your mother however explains that nothing was "stolen" but in fact she removed the toy to clean it. Your sibling didn't have all the information and their assumption and misplaced reaction has left you both feeling upset.

If your sibling had taking a moment to entertain other possibilities and asked a few questions before diving into a rage, a lot of pain and drama could have been avoided.

Seeking a wider perspective means gathering information about the reality of situation rather than simply believing that what you "think" is a fact. That coupled with a big picture view of the outcome you are seeking can help you avoid going down a road that leads to pain. If more people took the time to try to fully understand the situation and didn't jump to the most negative conclusion our world would be a different place.

However, it is important to understand that aiming to seek wider perspective does not mean staying in a harmful relationship or putting yourself in danger. In general knowing there is more to every story can help you direct your words and actions. But just because there is a good likelihood that you lack all the information, it is not a reason to let anyone hurt you.

It is important to be clear about this.

Just because a schoolyard bully may have been bullied himself is no cause to let the behaviour continue. In fact from a wider perspective it is all the more reason to ensure that that chain of events does not continue.

4. Is it Constructive or Destructive?

I can't speak for everyone but when I look at moments in my life that I experience true anger there are distinct qualities of it being either constructive or destructive. In moments of constructive anger, I feel like I had snapped out of a dream. Now fully awake, I am able to articulate myself clearly and speak (or yell) from a place deep within myself that is powerful and demands its due respect. The purpose of the anger in these cases was large in scope and the purpose went far beyond my own personal gain.

At times when I act out of anger that is destructive, my thoughts and words are muddled and I respond to my feelings with petty words and actions. Usually the situation feels very personal and painful.

Making these distinctions for yourself is an enormous help in determining how to work with anger. Constructive anger can be the catalyst to move you forward. Destructive anger needs another outlet and may be better used to fuel a creative project like a song or work of art.

Anger is a real response to something happening that needs to be investigated and respected. As yogis working towards being more conscious human beings, we need to face it head on, not stuff it down or pretend it isn't there. In Chinese Medicine, no emotion is inherently bad, it all depends on how gracefully we direct and allow them to pass through and move us forward.

Metal

"At no other time (than autumn) does the earth let itself be inhaled in one smell, the ripe earth; in a smell that is in no way inferior to the smell of the sea, bitter where it borders on taste, and more honey sweet where you feel it touching the first sounds. Containing depth within itself, darkness, something of the grave almost."
~ **Rainer Maria Rilke**, *Letters on Cézanne*

Metal: Fall in the City

The wind from the ocean contains a noticeable chill today as I walk through the park. From here I can see the water on Boston harbour. It looks choppy and uninviting and I bundle up my jacket in protest. Even in the middle of the city, against the backdrop of the tall grey buildings, the fall leaves are glorious. They seem to radiate their beauty fully today, offering one last show of colour before the snow arrives and wraps the city in white. The sunlight dances in and out between the grey clouds as I wander the same route I have walked alone nearly every day since I moved to Boston.

Today I am walking with only a slight limp and no more than a whisper of pain, though a few months ago I could barely walk at all. It had started slowly, probably the side effect of a cold I didn't take care of. A slight puffy discomfort around one knee spiralled into full blown swelling and chronic pain throughout my body. One specialist told me I would end up in a wheelchair within six months. I was frightened and devastated. This sudden physical barrier threw everything in my life into chaos and uncertainty.

How could I continue to run two businesses that were physically and emotionally demanding if I could barely climb the stairs to my office or studio?

Newly engaged, I worried that if continued to deteriorate quickly my partner might not want to take on the burden of looking after me. Who would want to marry someone if they could barely look after themselves?

Regardless of my fears, when I got sick, I had to face the fact that my current way of life wasn't going to cut it in my new reality of physical limitation. My loving partner urged me to make a significant change and move, at least temporarily, to Boston where he could care for me daily while I got some rest and perspective. Though I fought it at first, eventually it became clear that it was time to let go and surrender. I closed my clinic, said goodbye to my family, friends, and students and moved not only to be with my partner, but to be with myself.

It wasn't easy. I grieved the loss of the familiar and the safe, along with all the other relationships that confirmed who I was in the world. But I trusted that only by letting go could I build the next chapter with more space and care for that which is most important in life, for that which is most important to me.

The aroma of dry leaves and soggy earth pulls me back into the park. I turn towards my new home and pause to admire the trees one last time, grateful that I am here.

Metal

The Metal element is by far the most challenging of the Five Elements for yogis to grasp. Metal doesn't have the same clear symbols in nature the way the other elements do and that makes it difficult for people to make an intuitive connection. Metal represents the rocks and minerals found in the earth; they are the bones of our planet, and our bodies, hidden beneath the surface. As a physical structure, Metal is the body's armour (the skin) deciding what to take in and what to keep out. Metal is also a key to help us decide what to let go of whether it be physical (as seen in the exhalation and elimination of waste), emotional, or spiritual. This element is found in the fall breeze, the sound of weeping, and the dignity of the warrior.

The Season of Metal: Autumn

Metal corresponds to autumn. Fall is the time of the final harvest when the last crops that began to grow in the spring and flourish throughout the summer are finally collected. The type of food in abundance at this time of year tends to be hearty with a longer storage life than summer fruits and vegetables, nourishing us through the winter. Arriving well past the summer solstice, the fall is more yin in nature acting as a buffer between summer and winter. The autumn months offer time to prepare our resources and begin to conserve energy to survive the winter. The crisp cool air of this beautiful season and the graceful falling of leaves is a reminder that nothing in life is permanent and even the most perfect summer must come to an end in order to give way to new possibilities in the spring.

Fall is a magical and important time for the Elemental yogi. After the warmth and expansion of the summer, autumn allows you to reconnect to your practice and integrate all the breakthroughs the heat may have afforded.

The Organs

Metal is represented in the body in a number of ways. The bones, which are the last to dissolve after we die are one of the most energetically yin structures in the body and are Metal in nature. However, the physical organs of Metal are the Lungs (often referred to as the singular "Lung" in Chinese Medicine) and the Large Intestine.

Metal Yin: The Lung(s) - The Prime Minister

Often called the "tender organ" the Lung official represents the yin aspect of Metal in the body. The lungs are located close to the surface and are therefore more vulnerable than other vital organs. Their main function in our physical body is to take in air (that which is needed for life) and expel carbon dioxide (letting go of that which is no longer needed). Like the dutiful public servant in the opening fairytale of the book, the Lungs work for the greater good, supporting life and keeping nothing for themselves.

Lung energy holds the role of the Prime Minister. The Prime Minister works closely with the Empress (the Heart) and is in charge of making the practical arrangements and adjustments so that each of the officials receive what they need to do their jobs and realize the potential of the

Empire. The Lung/Prime Minster therefore controls the body's qi. Just as nations fall into chaos if they lack a rational and functional leader to keep things running smoothly, without healthy Lung energy the body could not function.

Metal Yang: The Large Intestine - The Transportation Official

In the Western medical model of the body the Large Intestine is an important organ in the digestive process. Interestingly, in Chinese Medicine many of the functions of this organ are attributed to Spleen energy. However, in both systems the Large Intestine has the responsibility of absorbing any last nutrients that have been sent there from the Small Intestine and moving waste out of the body.

The position held by the Large Intestine in our mythical Empire is that of transportation official. Just as you don't notice the intricate roadways and traffic signals until there is a problem, the Large Intestine plays a key role in our daily life even if it doesn't get much credit. When something goes awry in the transportation system traffic jams occur and can throw off the entire day. This interruption creates frustration and bad moods in the populace. Similarly, anyone who has suffered major issues with digestion and elimination can tell you how difficult it is to live with a disruption in this important bodily process that the rest of us take for granted.

Metal Themes

Valuing What Is Important in Life

The diamond is among the hardest materials on Earth and by its price tag you could assume it is a "rare gem." Many cultures have assigned great worth to these stones and have made them popular mainstays as expressions of love and devotion. Surprisingly diamonds are quite common, making them a perfect metaphor for much of what we have culturally stamped as "valuable." Once enough people deem something rare, stunning, or symbolic of "the good life," that object is assigned a high value whether or not it innately deserves this special esteem.

While money is not the only way in which we determine value, it is one of the most prevalent in our current culture and attaching a dollar amount to an object or experience tells us about its worth. For example, a rare luxury car or a famous designer's last gown would both fetch a high price.

But if suddenly the luxury car company mass produced the once rare vehicle and the designer sold her patent to a department store, the "special" factor would be lost and the value would plummet.

When we believe that something is special we treasure it. If you treasure music for instance, you can easily justify spending the time, energy, and money on years of lessons because it is aligned with your value system. If music is special and meaningful to you then the cost of working with a teacher and the hours spent practicing could not be better spent.

As a yogi you have probably invested a lot of time and effort on your mat, as well as money to take classes; gone on retreats; or taken a teacher training. Something about the practice inspires you and makes you feel the way you want to feel, so the time and energy are worth it.

Chinese Medicine is very tuned in to the amount of qi, or energy, each of us has. Although the Water element is the most connected with appropriate use of our resources and personal longevity, each element contributes to this dynamic in its own way. The health of Metal energy is important in how you use your inner resources: if this element is harmonized you can see clearly what is worthy of your time and energy. If however Metal is tarnished or diseased, you risk ascribing value to objects and relationships that are not healthy or worthy of your qi. Working with Metal, you will learn to distinguish the valuable from the frivolous, the worthy from the unworthy.

When what is important becomes clear you can decide how best to use your personal resources. Your time, energy, and money will be invested only in things you truly value.

Self-Worth

Metal, sensitive to what you treasure, is deeply connected to your self-worth. If you are someone who values your mind, body, and spirit, you likely express that dignity in how you interact with the world. If however you have been taught that you are not special or valuable, you may compensate by building yourself a metaphorical suit of armour to hide behind.

We can all do this in countless ways when we feel insecure. We might use status symbols, such as expensive clothing or shiny accessories, to try and distract the world from our personally perceived flaws. We might name-drop, talking about the important people we know, or make a point to wax on about interesting things we've done, coming off as vapid and superficial.

If you are someone who lacks self-worth you may tend to conceal your true thoughts and feelings in an effort to be more likable, and then have a hard time opening up in relationships for fear that your flaws far outweigh your good qualities. Ironically when you don't have a healthy sense of self-worth, you will search for validation from the outside world.

Here a vicious cycle begins.

You may project a certain mask or persona to the world in hopes of getting the positive feedback you desire. If you don't get the response you seek, it drives you to put up more walls against the world and add new layers to your mask. When positive feedback does come, it doesn't satisfy you because it was an insincere version of yourself that "fooled" the world into offering you praise. Convinced that no one could love or respect the person that you are, you hide behind your mask until it becomes too thick for even the most compassionate person to penetrate.

It is part of the human experience to wear different hats and masks as our situations and comfort levels change, but if it becomes the norm, personal dignity becomes scarce. Harmonizing the Metal element allows you to recognize and celebrate the unique combination of energy, experience, and circumstances that have shaped you, and enables you to move through the world with a sense of self-worth that doesn't need external validation.

Letting Go

Just as leaves fall from the trees in autumn, so too must each one of us release aspects of life that no longer fit who we are. We must metaphorically exhale the things that have run their course if we want to be able to inhale the fresh and new opportunities of life. This can happen at several levels from the mundane to the deeply spiritual.

Letting go serves an important practical purpose. We take in what we need—air, food, water—and let go of what we don't need in order to make room for the next wave of life-giving fuel for the body. A healthy body doesn't ponder whether or not to exhale, fearing that the next inhalation may not come, the body trusts that only by letting go will it receive what it needs from the next breath.

Practical Letting Go

Beyond the body, however, letting go may be more complicated, especially when it comes to the physical clutter of our daily lives. It is easy to accumulate a lot of "stuff"—everything from overflowing email accounts to mystery boxes filling up storage space or clothes that haven't been worn in years bursting out of a closet. The organization industry is booming right now and for good reason. Most of us have way too much that we don't need and don't enjoy.

As a yoga practitioner you probably already know that the external and internal reflect one another. It is easier to be productive at work if your desk is neat and your workspace is inviting and inspiring. You may on the other hand notice what a turn off it is to wade through a messy or overpacked store when you are shopping.

While spring may be the traditional time to clean and freshen up your surroundings, an autumn decluttering of your life is a lovely way to make use of the new seasonal energy and let go of any residual mental, physical, and emotional clutter.

Emotional Letting Go

Once you begin letting go, you may feel inspired to go deeper with this practice and declutter old habits and emotions that are stagnating your mind and body. You might find the most impactful way to do this starts with handling the negativity that is orbiting your life. Negative emotions are natural and it would be naive to expect a life where you never encounter them. One day you wake up in a bad mood. Another day a friend or family member is suffering and their pain affects you. Denying your real and valid emotions when you are dealing with a primarily negative situation is not my suggestion.

The negativity purge I am suggesting aims at getting rid of the junk that sneaks through your filters and creates low-grade stress and anxiety. Personally, when I started taking this inner work seriously a few years ago I realized that the most precious commodity I have is my time and energy. I took stock of how I was spending these valuable things and it resulted in backing away from people who only reached out to me when they had a problem or used our time "together" to talk only about themselves.

Knowing I could never get my precious time back, I stopped giving it to people who constantly gossiped about their other friends or made a habit of complaining. Not surprisingly, the less time I spent around negative people, the less negative my own thoughts and behaviours became. While it may seem harsh at first to examine other people in this way, the nature of healthy Metal is seeing situations in a rational way and protecting yourself from the influence of whatever is draining and stifling your inspiration.

Check out the exercises at the end of this chapter to help you as you let go of physical and emotional clutter.

Letting Go and Impermanence

Letting go of what is no longer needed is, of course, practically useful when it comes to material clutter and the resulting emotional health; spiritually, however, the process becomes even more profound. Learning this art is a functional reminder of the impermanent nature of life. Although we know change and loss is inevitable, most people operate within their lives as though the way things are is the way they will always be. In fact, it makes sense that you would assume that what you had yesterday will still be there tomorrow—your home, your job, your relationships. It would be too exhausting to worry that your life might be turned upside down with each new day, and it would create constant emotional turmoil to imagine your life without your most treasured loved ones, without your career, without your most fundamental physical and mental capacities. And yet in an instant everything can change.

Some people prefer to ignore this undeniable reality. When an unexpected loss occurs it shocks them to the core and can sometimes lead to deep long-term emotional and psychological issues. Spiritual practitioners tend to take another approach. Having observed that life is impermanent by its very nature, instead of holding on tightly to protect their bubble of valuable "stuff," they use the fact of impermanence as a lodestar. Impermanence offers an opportunity to be grateful and to never take for granted the health, relationships, and opportunities you are afforded in each moment.

Impermanence is a fact that invites you to stay present with the beauty of life more often, and to appreciate what is in front of you fully before it is gone.

Metal: On the Mat

It is no coincidence that yoga poses which create expansion through the chest or involve a deepening of the breath create an almost instantaneous, positive shift for the yoga practitioner. While many yogis love pranayama (breathing practice) and backbends, both of which seem to create more space through the front of the chest, others feel exposed and anxious during these postures.

By far one of the most important and symbolic yoga asanas for the Metal element is savasana, the corpse pose, the moment at the end of an asana session where you allow your body to completely let go. While many teachers glaze over savasana's traditional death symbolism, preferring to call it "final relaxation," the corpse-like stillness of this posture assists the student in a profound release and is meant to be a symbolic practice of the letting go we each must do at the end of life.

For a few precious moments there is space for you to take a break from your sometimes hectic life full of goals and effort and be completely free. This space prepares the yogi for more grace off the mat and serves as a reminder that this incarnation is precious and impermanent.

The Emotion of Metal: Grief

The nature of an ending may be orchestrated and logical, such as the completion of a project that makes space for something new, or it may be sudden and unexpected, such as the death of a dear friend or the loss of a dream job. In either case, it is normal to grieve loss or mourn the end of a chapter in life.

As a Chinese Medicine practitioner one of the things I would constantly stress to my clients is that emotions are natural and each one has a healthy expression that provides the opportunity to transform. The same is true of grief, the emotion of Metal. And yet many people are confused about how to navigate the experience. Because we live in a world that is obsessed with "happiness," you may have been urged from a young age to paste on a smile and "cheer up," or to self-medicate at the first sign of sadness. You may have learned that grief is shameful even if it is in response to a painful and real loss.

Being restricted from expressing natural feelings of grief over life's changes in the long term can leave you feeling defensive and isolated. Healthy Metal energy becomes damaged. Stagnant, unexpressed grief can lead to deeper disruptions within a person, such as long-term depression, obsessive perfectionism, or even excessively superficial behaviour in order to avoid a meaningful connection to life for fear of the inevitable loss in the future.

The turnaround is that when you feel sadness over the end of something meaningful in your life, it indicates that you care very deeply. For instance, when a community grieves the death of a loved one together it can forge an immediate lifelong connection between people even if they are complete strangers. Grief can be cathartic as well as provide a platform for transformation and, in some cases, a redirection of purpose— life, grief reminds us, is undeniably uncertain. To help us from getting wrapped up in drama, frivolity, and wasting our days, Metal teaches us to use this precious life for something inspiring and beautiful.

Metal Constitution:
Amanda - The Professional Perfectionist

Amanda is a massage therapist and counsellor. She spends her days in sessions with people who tell her their problems, outline their emotional and physical injuries, and reveal their deepest secrets. Although she has a hard time admitting it, she is spectacular at both of her jobs. Her perfectionist nature compels her to work hard and, as a result, she has been recognized with awards in both fields.

Her clients describe her as a miracle worker. She listens deeply and reflects back to people what they most need in a way that cuts through their excuses. Her clients trust her because she is mindful, professional, and doesn't rush people to change faster than they are ready to. At the same time, Amanda doesn't let her clients off the hook once they commit to making changes for their health and well-being. She teaches others how to value themselves and their lives.

On the outside Amanda is well put together and to the outside observer seems slightly high-maintenance. She spends up to an hour each morning grooming her hair, applying the perfect make-up, and matching her accessories expertly to her outfit. Her attention to detail and her perfectionist streak extend to most aspects of her life and work, but where those tendrils don't reach, she falls to the other extreme. Amanda can't seem to keep her house tidy. She can't bear to part with any of her stuff just in case she might need it again in the future.

Amanda has many acquaintances in the different compartments of her life, but few close friends. Those who do get into her inner circle are treated like family and get to know the whole picture of who Amanda is. However if anyone from the inner circle hurts her deeply, she immediately shuts down and will cut them out in a heartbeat. Second chances do not come easily, if at all, and though the offending party may judge her as cold and unfeeling, it is really the coat of armour Amanda wears to shield herself from getting hurt again.

Someone with a Metal constitution, or Metal disharmony, can have trouble letting go. Metal types sometimes cry for almost no reason or lament an old loss or injury as though it happened yesterday. Others act stoic and guarded. They can also have the tendency to devalue themselves or search endlessly for external validation. Ironically, this insecurity can lead to highly superficial behaviour and the quest for validation may never end if Metal doesn't allow anyone beyond the gates to see them deeply enough to treasure.

Harmonious Metal people have a healthy sense of self-worth and dignity. They deal with the inevitable losses and endings in life with grace. To be with them when they grieve is to feel both beauty and love even in the midst of sorrow. They are also known for being masters of mirroring back the value and possibilities of those who are lucky enough to be near them. Like a diamond refracts and reflects light, this constitution seems to shine when inspiring others to utilize their deep potential and not waste a moment of this valuable and special life. Metal sees the beauty in the limited time and energy we are each afforded in this life and when fully powered can help ensure that there is more dignity in the world and that every day is treasured.

Metal Exercises:
Organizing Your Living & Working Space

The most obvious place to begin to let go of what is no longer needed is in your home and workspace. Autumn is the perfect season to get rid of things you don't need or love, but you can invoke the spirit of Metal at anytime of year when you need to declutter.

Here is a simple technique I often share and have found very useful:

Organized Living

Creating a living space you love turns your home into a true sanctuary and a place to rest and restore so you can be more present in your life. Spend 10-20 minutes each day decluttering one area of your living space. If you have more time, you can tackle an entire room, but it is best to start small because this can eat up your time quickly.

Here's the technique:

1) Take four bags or bins labeled: Trash, Recycle, Donate, Belongs Elsewhere.

2) Pick one area to declutter. Take out all the items in that space and place them on the floor. One by one go through each item asking if this is still useful and valued at this point in your life. Once you decide, place each item in its appropriate bag and put back anything that belongs where it started.

3) Immediately find the home of the "Belongs Elsewhere" items (seriously, do not wait on this one). You aren't finished until that bag is empty and everything is in its home.

4) Take out the trash and recycling so it isn't cluttering your living space. Once the donation bag is full give it away to a local charity or a friend in need.

After a major de-cluttering, put the finishing touches on by doing a deep clean. Personally, after spending a lot of time getting rid of unwanted artifacts from my past the last thing I feel like doing is a deep clean (actually I don't get joy out of cleaning anytime). Instead, I hire someone to come and clean my home a day or two after the planned tidying session.

Letting Go of Negativity

The more work you do to uncover what is most valuable in your life the more aware you will become of the unhealthy relationships you have. In many cases, with a little bit of work certain relationships can grow, if both you and the other person are willing to shift the way you interact. If however you find yourself in relationships that feel one-sided or you cringe when certain people reach out, it is time to reexamine your involvement.

Write down the following:

- Who is the most optimistic and inspired person in your life?

- What makes them that way? Do they have a special practice or outlook? (If you don't know, ask them and find out)

- How do you feel when you are around them?

- Who is the most negative person in your life?

- What makes them that way? Do you know of a certain experience that allowed them to draw negative conclusions about the world?

- How do you feel when you are around them?

If these two people are the extremes of the spectrum, where do most of your close friends and family members (i.e. the people you probably spend the most time with) fall?

The surprising insight that many of my student have when completing this exercise is that they often spend more time and energy on the negative people on the spectrum than they realized or were comfortable with. With that information you can decide how to proceed in your life and when to perhaps let go of relationships that have run their course.

Earth

"Heaven is under our feet as well as over our heads."
~ **Henry David Thoreau,** *Walden*

Can I Do This?

It is the middle of the night and like every night in the past few months I am lying in bed wide awake. I can hear the soft breathing of my sleeping husband asleep beside me, a sharp contrast to the tiny being doing somersaults in my womb. I mentally tell her that here on the outside we sleep at night, but the only response is a kick to my ribs.

Many women claim they love being pregnant and that during pregnancy they feel filled with true purpose. These natural nurturers always wanted to parent a child, whereas I, more than halfway through my pregnancy, am still convinced I am not cut out for the job.

It's not that I don't love children.

It's just that I didn't expect this process that billions of women go through to feel so foreign. Instead of feeling like pregnancy is natural, I feel like my body is being hijacked and I have no control.

My deep worry is that I won't be able to take care of my daughter as well as other mothers care for their children. I haven't always done a great job nurturing myself and it makes me wonder: If I can't adequately nurture myself, how will I care for a being that will depend on me for her every need?

I went through a health crisis not long ago. Mysterious joint pain and swelling spread like wildfire throughout my entire body. Some days I could barely walk and although I have been living pain free for some time since, my doctor warned me that if my condition was a type of arthritis I may experience a major flare-up after giving birth.

The looming possibility that I might not be able to hold and care for my daughter after she is born is a thought that haunts me even though there is nothing I can do to change what may happen.

The only relief from this worry is the support and assurance I receive from my husband. Since the wild ride of pregnancy began, he has been with me for nearly every appointment, cooked meal after meal trying to find something I could stomach, and comforted me through the fears, questions, and inevitable physical discomforts. While my ability to nurture is still unknown, his has blossomed.

The tiny soccer player in my belly takes a few more shots and then starts to quiet down. Although it is still some time before my mind follows suit, the stream of thoughts finally run their course. I am lulled back to sleep by the sound of my husband breathing, aware that my unborn child and I have all the support we need.

Earth

Earth is not only one of the Five elements, it is the ground on which we stand and the foundation of life. It is no wonder why so many cultures give the mother archetype to this element. We depend on the multitude of offerings she provides. Without Earth the other elements would have no home to centralize around.

In the body Earth is represented by the muscles and through digestion the organs receive the ingredients to produce and move qi throughout the body. When this element thrives in nature it yields the food we need and the support system at the basis of all life on the planet. However natural disasters, such as earthquakes, can have drastic and deadly consequences. Similarly when overused or treated poorly, the land we rely on can become toxic and barren. The Earth element gives so much that it is easy to take its gifts for granted, but without the essential support of Earth we could not exist.

The Season of Earth:
Late Summer or the In-Between Times

The season governed by the Earth element depends on what school of Chinese Medicine philosophy you subscribe to. Interestingly none connects Earth to any of the traditional four seasons. One school teaches that the Earth element rules late summer (usually the final six weeks before autumn). This specific time of year holds the abundance of the summer harvest. Fields overflow with succulent summer crops and this bounty continues into the fall. The days are no longer stifling and hot but the weather is still beautiful. There is also a clear sense that autumn is just around the corner. Those who are in tune with the seasons will notice a shift that stirs the senses and insists you give special attention to those final, precious days of summer and enjoy their fleeting beauty.

Other theories regard the season of Earth not as a season at all but as the transition period between each of the four distinct seasons. In this model, the final few weeks of fall, winter, spring, and summer are all governed by Earth energy.

When I was an acupuncturist and herbal practitioner, the transition between the seasons was a popular time for clients to come to me seeking help with sleep or seasonal illness as their bodies adjusted to fluctuating temperatures and varying degrees of daylight. Perhaps you have noticed that the change in seasons creates ripples and upheaval in your schedule. Working with the Earth element during those times can be useful in helping to smooth out the transition.

The Organs

Earth Yin: The Spleen - The Minister of Food

In Chinese Medicine the Spleen and Stomach are a pair that work together closely. Like many organs in Chinese Medicine, the function of the Spleen is much different in this theory than in Western physiology. For the purposes of Elemental yin yang thinking, the Spleen energy is the Minister of Food. This official has the vital job of making sure each region of the Empire has enough quality sustenance and energy. In times of famine a qualified Minister of Food needs to ration supplies and extract the energy of every last useful morsel to be distributed it to those who need it most.

When the Spleen is overwhelmed there can be issues with fatigue, bloating, and dampness collecting in pockets of the body (like the joint swelling I described at the beginning of this chapter) among other things.

The healthy Spleen is in charge, transforming nutrients from food and drink into qi and blood and moving it throughout the body and helping to pass along waste towards its final destination.

Earth Yang: The Stomach - The Food Processing Plant

The Spleen and Stomach are closely linked: if the Spleen is the Minister of Food than the Stomach acts as the food processing plant. All the food and drink one ingests makes its way to this processing centre where it undergoes the first stage of being broken down. The Stomach ripens and rottens food to make it easier for the Spleen to work with and distribute.

Earth Themes

From Collaboration to Devotional Love

The body depends on Earth organs collaborating to transform outside food into useful energy. This is just one of the most basic ways humans depend on a close relationship between ourselves and the world we are part of. Our miraculous bodies are only designed to work within a specific exterior environment that provides the foundation of life. If the planet's temperature or gravitational field were to change even slightly, Earth would be uninhabitable.

Our ability to thrive exists further by the grace of collaboration with other humans in both personal and impersonal ways. The fact that I can sit and write these words on a computer that contains countless inventions and innovations within its casing, have those words printed into a book so that you, with your intellect and understanding, can read and interpret their meaning is truly incredible.

How many millions of people over the span of human existence contributed to the exchange we are having as author and reader in this very moment?

Human collaboration has advanced everything in culture from music and art to medicine and technology. As such, our lives are impersonally intertwined more deeply than we know.

From birth we depend on our caregivers to provide food and shelter, and to protect and teach us how to survive in the world. When I became a mother, all the worry and fear I'd had about not being up to the task evaporated and was replaced with both a profound love and an overwhelming sense of responsibility toward my child, a familiar experience of every parent. Without knowing anything about my daughter—her preferences, her thoughts, her feelings, who she will grow up to be—I loved her instantly.

When she was placed on my chest just seconds after she was born, a type of love hit me that I can only describe as blind devotion. Without a thought, I was able to drop whatever I was doing to feed and change this tiny being. I held her when she cried no matter what time of day or night.

In the baby/parent relationship, parents give endlessly to their child, sacrificing sleep and setting aside aspects of their former lifestyle all to take on their new role as nurturer. This type of love and devotion is an expression of Earth. While love is typically a Fire theme, this unique kind of love that puts the needs of another before the desires of the self is governed by Earth. My relationship with my child is one where I give freely whatever I can but there is no conscious reciprocity on her part. It is no wonder why an affectionate name for our planet is Mother Earth. It's the element that gives.

Nurturing Others Demands Self-Care

When I was in school studying Chinese Medicine, the topic of self-care was highlighted often. We were encouraged to employ a wide array of techniques to help keep ourselves open, healthy, and available for our patients. While I agreed with this in theory, and even preached the importance of self-care, in reality I went through years subtly neglecting my need for sleep, consistent nutrition, and regular time off. Part of me felt self-indulgent if I took a day off just because I was feeling low energy, or if I didn't take on an extra client or class just because my day was "a little full."

In the opening reflection for both Earth and Metal, I shared how undermining my own health and well-being began a painful dance with burnout and illness. I learned the hard way what happens if you try to support and nurture others without taking care of yourself at the same time. After years of pushing too hard and saying yes to every demand on my time and energy my health took a downward spiral.

The Earth element has a special relationship with the kind of physical "dampness" I experienced in my joints. Like a crop field that can't absorb nutrients and fresh water, this stagnation sat in the pockets of my body. I was in near constant pain with severely limited mobility.

The ironic lesson here is that by not caring for myself, I lost touch with why I was caring for others, and subsequently burnt out. Luckily, Elemental Yoga and its corresponding philosophy of using both yin and yang types of self-care were instrumental as I moved forward towards a more harmonious approach to life.

The exercises at the end of this chapter will help you learn to rethink how you nurture yourself so that you can better care for the important things in your life.

Integrity

The Earth element is the central point around which the other elements converge. Without Earth, there would be no ground from which Wood could grow. There would be no boundaries to contain the Waters of the oceans, lakes, and rivers. There would be no fuel nor foundation for Fire to burn upon and Metal would have nothing to imbue with its nutrients. Earth is the mother, the source of life that carries us through the stages of development and it is where we return at the end of our days.

Because Earth is a converging point, it is assigned the theme of integrity in Elemental Yin Yang Yoga. Having integrity is one of the most important qualities a spiritual seeker can cultivate. Being able to remain whole and undivided by supporting your words with appropriate actions and vice versa is a powerful practice. A person with integrity doesn't need to ruminate over the way they project themselves in the world. They don't have to stay vigilant in making sure they project the "correct" version depending on the situation and who is there. Instead they are free to use their qi in service of working toward their dreams—their mind, body, and soul are unified and grounded in their overarching purpose.

Earth: On the Mat

According to Chinese Medicine, Earth governs the muscles so when working with this element, any postures that strengthen the body or bear the body's weight could be generally considered Earth by their nature. More specifically however the Earth element works closely with the digestive organs and the stabilizing core muscles. The "core" is more than just the abdominals in this instance. It is the muscle group that collaborates while holding an elbow plank or lifting something heavy from the ground and bracing through your body's centre. Twists are also Earth in nature because they squeeze and move the centre of the body.

The process of learning how to make your practice more holistic is another way to gain the wisdom of Earth on the mat. Elemental Yin Yang Yoga offers the practitioner an opportunity to both build strength and release tension.

During the yang portion of practice, the yogi first spends time developing physical intelligence within the laboratory of the body. That work is then integrated while nourishing yourself physically, mentally and emotionally in the yin postures.

It is the best of two asana worlds and even those with strong preferences on pace of practice or a particular style can enjoy the yoga they gravitate to while simultaneously expanding their horizons.

The Emotion of Earth: Rumination

The emotion associated with the Earth element varies slightly between schools of Chinese philosophy, but in Elemental Yin Yang Yoga the state associated with this element is worry or rumination. At its root, worry and overthinking are a testament to our ability as humans to discern and consider the impact of different paths we might take.

In order to fixate on a thought or situation, several highly advanced processes are occurring. For a person to overthink, they must have the capacity to recall and process the past, weigh its impact on the present, and imagine different possible futures. There is also an ability to review and interpret information from several sources and to solve problems among other things.

Another source of worry comes from being a sensitive, caring individual. The fact that humans at this stage of evolution have the ability to care enough about people and the world around them is truly remarkable. However when thinking becomes excessive it can be a primary cause for anxiety and stress.

As a culture we have normalized worry and its side effects can have drastic consequences on our collective health as a species. When there is an Earth disharmony, you will find yourself more prone to overthinking and replaying distressing thoughts to the point of obsession.

The process usually begins innocently.

Imagine you are given an interesting job opportunity in a city far from where you live. With this life-altering decision placed in front of you, the rational thing to do is to take time to consider the options so you can make the best move possible. After mulling it over, you make a list of the pros and cons attached to each direction and think through the myriad of possible outcomes. While you hoped doing this would make the choice clear, now you feel more overwhelmed by all the "what if's" attached to the job.

What if the job isn't as good as your current one?

What if your new relationship can't handle the distance and you break up?

What if you don't take this new job and then get laid off in a few months?

Feeling more unsure than when you first started, you seek outside advice. You ask your sister, your friends, your coworkers, and anyone else who will listen. However the feedback you get makes things worse. Your sister and your best friend completely disagree on what course to follow and now, stuck, you are no closer to moving forward. While other elemental energies are at play in this scenario, the replaying of the same ideas and concerns over and over again without action are an Earth issue.

Worry and overthinking can lead to paralyzing anxiety, stress, and exhaustion. The mental gymnastics of replaying the same situation over and over again in your mind, whether it is a past event that you wish hadn't happened or a situation you worry may occur in the future, consumes a tremendous amount of your inner resources. In my story at the beginning of this chapter, I described how my mind ran wild about how my life would change after my daughter was born. As much as this is perfectly natural, in hindsight I wish I employed the tools of yoga and meditation more often to help divert that energy to other things.

Many people similarly waste their mental capacities fruitlessly reviewing a past they can't change and planning their responses and reactions for the unknowable future. They miss the opportunity to use their precious time and incredible mind to respond to what is in front of them one thing at a time. It is like worrying before a big exam about how hard it is going to be and what you will do with your life after you fail, instead of just studying for it as best as you can.

Your mind is an amazing tool but it can only work for you in the way you train it to. Training the mind on the mat and the meditation cushion provides a respite from our fast paced, overstimulating world. Through learning how to objectify and get space from the source of your rumination you have more opportunity to keep the positive attributes of deep thought, care, and intelligence without the harmful effects of long-term stress.

The Earth Constitution:
Angela - The Nurturer

When you first meet Angela, you will be taken by her big beautiful eyes and her curvy figure. Like a living Botticelli, Angela is the archetypal Earth Mama. Her speaking voice is a soothing song and you can't help but feel comforted by her presence. Although she has just two children of her own, her house is constantly full of kids and she welcomes them all. Her kindness doesn't stop there. She makes time to connect with people in all pockets of her life paying special attention to those who live far from their family. Angela makes everyone feel included and cared for, from her clients and coworkers to her best friends.

While Angela spends a great deal of energy nurturing others, she doesn't spend nearly enough looking after herself. She will neglect sleep and meal times putting other priorities ahead of her own. Being so overly helpful at work means her boss doesn't hesitate to ask her to meet more restrictive deadlines than her colleagues. And although she knows she is being taken advantage of, she dislikes conflict or feeling like she has let anyone down so she simply does the extra work.

Apart from work, Angela struggles occasionally with feelings of resentment. While her generosity is authentic she wishes sometimes that others would go the extra mile to help her even though she has a hard time asking for support. Because she doesn't know how to ask, her loved ones think she doesn't need them as much as they need her and easily miss the subtle signs that she needs more nourishment from them.

Earth constitutions and those with an Earth disharmony may find that they give more than they receive and struggle silently with resentment, worry and anxiety. Although any constitution can experience these emotions, some Earth types manage anxiety by focusing it outward, giving their advice and opinions to others even when it isn't asked for.

Excessive Earth people may seem overbearing because they project their worries on to their friends and family as a tactic to deal with their own unresolved anxiety. When they give something they expect to receive something of equal or greater value back from the recipient. This can lead to disappointment when these expectations aren't met.

A deficient Earth type, on the other hand, may support others to their own detriment. Bending over backwards to make the people in their life happy may result in them being taken advantage of or used like a doormat. These types may internalize their feelings because they don't want to "put anyone else out."

A harmonized Earth type knows how to take care of their own needs while nurturing others. They know that the only way to truly extend their generosity is as a gift that has no strings attached and no repayment needed. This brilliant Earth type knows how to use their abundance and energy on things they can change and doesn't get ruffled by things they can't control. Healthy Earth energy operates with as much integrity as possible; they say what they mean, mean what they say, and have the trust and confidence of those around them.

Earth Exercise: Self-Care

When I speak with yoga students about their biggest challenges surrounding the practice, by far the most common is making time to get on the mat. The demands of a hectic schedule can pull even the most dedicated yogi's focus away from the mat. Even though we know yoga improves everything from our energy to our outlook on life, many people experience feelings of guilt when they make time for their yoga practice over other things.

While a daily practice may not be in the cards for everyone, I always ask my students to consider that when we make the space in life for quality self-care, the effects trickle outward into the world. Personally, if I have not prioritized my yoga and meditation practice, I land in a bad mood much more easily than when I have honoured my need for the space and replenishment those practices provide. It is profoundly simple. When I am uptight and low energy I am not going to operate from the very best I have to offer. When I am well-rested and refuelled I tend to be more patient, supportive and able to express the best I have to offer the world.

Yin and Yang Self-Care

When you hear the phrase "self-care", warm baths or buying yourself flowers may come to mind. But self-care means so much more.

While one dimension of self-care is the more traditional version (the warm baths and flowers route). This is would be considered a yin form as it is nurturing and enveloping. Yin self-care is what the person who loves you most in the world does for you when you are having a rough day or feeling sick, encircling you with kindness and support.

Another aspect of self-care that is often overlooked is the yang dimension. It's the type of care that a coach or mentor might deliver. While still Earth by the nature of its overall goal, this type of positivity challenges you to express your highest potential. Yang self-care doesn't let you eat a bag of cookies on the sofa while you binge watch a bad t.v. series, it is the part of you that gets you up and out to the gym or to yoga.

Yin self-care is nurturing and recharging.

Yang self-care is inspiring and developmental.

Here are some examples to help you further distinguish the two:

Yin Self Care:

- Go to bed early so you can get a full 7-8 hrs of sleep

- Take a tech break, free from phone calls and email

- Spend time with loved ones enjoying a long meal

- Read a novel

Yang Self Care

- Get up early in the morning to do your yoga practice

- Spend a day pushing through outstanding work so you can relax on the weekend

- Spend time with loved ones working out, or doing some healthy activity

- Learn a new skill or hobby that challenges your intellect and perspective

Learn to cultivate both types of self-care in your life even if one comes easier than the other because they are each extremely important to our health and well-being.

What Kind of Self-Care do I Need?

As human beings, it is important to be aware that we have the tendency to favour one type of self-care over the other. Those who favour yin self-care tend to judge yang forms as being too aggressive or busy and therefore not self-care at all. Those who lean more towards yang self-care may in turn see yin forms as being lazy and indulgent. Knowing that you probably have a preference it is important to build the skill to self-assess what you truly need in a given situation rather than act based on your past habits.

If you have worked a 50+ hour week and slept no more than 6 hours each night, some Yin self-care is in order.

If things have been light in your schedule but you still feel underlying stress or the need for something more, a dose of yang is the fire you need.

There is no hard and fast rule to determine what your self-care regime might include, but I will offer a few simple guidelines that apply to both Yin and Yang self-care.

1. If it doesn't fuel you or nourish you, it isn't self-care.

2. Self-care means you do it for yourself. While asking for help or support is wonderful, self-care should be empowering and something you can do for yourself with as little reliance anywhere else as possible.

3. Self-care is something you look forward to. If you don't enjoy a deep benefit, it won't fuel or nourish you.

4. Self-care results in health and vitality. Self-care doesn't mean going out and eating a 3-layer cake or drinking excessively. Never use "self-care" to justify behaviour that is harmful to you or anyone else.

5. Self-care is necessary to your well-being, take it seriously.

Elemental
Asanas

Before You Begin

Many books have been written on the practice, science and art of physical (Hatha) yoga. There are schools all over the world, each with their own strong opinions on alignment, asana anatomy and the ideal way to sequence a yoga practice. While there are key principles that help to define what Elemental Yin Yang Yoga is and how yogis might use it, the pages that follow provide suggestions for how the yoga student or teacher might use the postures as a metaphor to work with certain themes from the Five Elements.

Why No Points and Meridians?

While occasionally there are notes about the main energetic pathways (or meridians), I deliberately do not focus on posture anatomy or moving qi through these channels or to point locations.

It is my firm belief that specific work around moving qi in the meridians and specific points be done in-person with a highly qualified Taiji or Qigong teacher or in a session with a licensed acupuncturist who has studied Chinese Medicine closely for years.

When I worked as a clinical acupuncturist, I witnessed how powerful these tools are. While the points and meridians can be helpful, using them without personal guidance and the years it takes to understand, diagnose and treat issues of the body, mind and spirit is like drilling into the water pipeline to get a glass of water instead of simply turning on the tap. You will get your glass of water, but you might find yourself dealing with much more than you can handle.

Unlike a painkiller that can be taken by almost anyone for who is dealing with pain, the points work in conjunction with one another and in combination with the individual's constitution and the way that a disease or disharmony is manifesting. It is overly simplistic to say that a certain point is used for stomach pain and another is for headaches. In Chinese Medicine, the practitioner needs to know if a stomach pain or headache is from: over-eating, under-eating, a certain food, a suspected external pathogenic invasion, heat or dampness to name a few of the many possibilities.

Because the way an individual should be treated using the system of Chinese Medicine and the acupoints is complex, I do not feel that a public yoga class is the right setting to work specifically trying to stimulate points along the meridians. A point that might be helpful in building the energy of one person could drain another.

If you are interested in doing qi and point work at a deep level, seek out a trained Chinese Medicine professional and give yourself the gift of that holistic approach.

This isn't to say that Elemental Yin Yang Yoga doesn't deal with the channels and points however. The beauty of this style is that simply doing a yoga practice is often enough for students to get the benefit of moving energy around the body and experience a naturally corrected flow of qi, without doing specific work with the meridians or acupoints.

Elemental Yin Yang Yoga: A Ritual of Movement

Setting-up For Practice

Here are some tips to help you set up a solid home practice from my course Yin Yang Yoga: Build Your Home Practice.

Learn more at:
www.udemy.com/yin-yang-yoga-build-your-home-practice

1. Make Space and Set the Mood

Before you begin your practice, make sure you have everything you need: your mat, your blocks and clothing appropriate for your environment and the temperature.

At a bare minimum, you need enough level, uncluttered surface area immediately surrounding your mat to move on. In an ideal situation, you should set up the space to be beautiful, inspirational and alive. The space and mood of your setting then becomes an extension of your practice and makes you feel joyful and ready to have the best practice possible.

Be rigid about being comfortable enough to let go on the mat. This is so important. One might think yoga in a forest at twilight is going to be blissful…and for the mosquitoes eating you alive, it just might be. Find a place to practice, whether it's indoors or outdoors, that isn't going to pull your focus off the mat for any reason.

Be flexible about where you practice if options are limited.
Before I became a professional yoga teacher, I used to tour manage a band. Living on the road for weeks at a time meant that I sometimes had to practice yoga during a sound check on the concrete floor of whatever bar or theatre we were going to play in that night. It taught me to be flexible about my surroundings and stretch myself to be creative about where I practiced when the situation wasn't ideal.

2. Defend Your Time

This is a big one and often the most challenging. If you live in a space with other people, make sure they know that for the amount of time you set aside, you are not to be interrupted.

Be flexible because defending your time also means that you are being reasonable with it. If you live other people (especially with young children), it may be best to wait until no one is home or things are quiet during your yoga session so your attention isn't being pulled outside the four corners of your mat.

If that isn't possible, find a time in the early morning or later at night when life is less busy. Do what you can with the time and space you have, but don't give up on practicing just because the timing isn't perfect.

Be rigid about unplugging completely for the full duration of your session. Turn off anything that rings or buzzes. Any teacher worth their salt would be horrified if you answered a phone call during class. Show yourself and your home practice the same respect. Your emails, texts and voicemails will be there waiting for you when you are finished and you will be much better equipped to deal with them after an uninterrupted yoga session.

3. Get Involved With Your Practice

In order to make your home practice come alive, you need to be interested and involved in the process of learning more about Yoga. Get your hands on as much reading material and interactive resources as your time and wallet allow. Taking workshops and regular classes and even private one-on-one lessons are all great ways to fuel your budding home practice.

Be rigid about following what excites you the most. When I began yoga, I was very shy about approaching my favourite instructors and asking them questions or for help with my practice. In hindsight, I can see clearly how limiting that lack of direct involvement was. As a teacher, I love students who are passionate enough about their practice to regularly engage with me in person or on our Yin Yang Yoga Facebook page.

Join the conversation:
www.facebook.com/groups/elementalyoga

Be flexible about where you get resources. We are lucky enough to live in a world where you can take private classes in-person and online. There is almost nothing standing in the way of getting all the help and support you need to practice, so get involved with your practice whether it happens at home or in the studio.

Above all else, treat your home practice with the same respect and care you would if you were practicing yoga at your favourite studio with your own teacher and enjoy it!

Principles of Elemental Yin Yang Yoga

Why Yang Flow Before Yin Postures?

The yang flow comes before the long-held yin poses. Although in some schools of yoga, yin is practiced without any warming of the muscles (i.e. before the yang flow), over the years I have found this to be less optimal for two reasons.

The first is physical. The average person who lives life moving from their seat in the car, to their desk chair at work, to their sofa at night, may not have the mobility to jump into a long held posture that puts stress on their joints, tendons and ligaments without first warming up. Those who are hyper-mobile on the other hand probably may need to avoid "opening" themselves further and thus long-held postures in a cold body may further strain or stretch areas that truly will not benefit the practitioner in the long run.

Practicing a yang flow before any long-held yin postures is also a way I help to "warm up" awareness and the tools my students need in order to let go. In our fast paced culture it can be difficult to expect a room full of people to walk in the door, unroll their mat and be still in postures for a long period of time. Many students need some time to flush the frantic energy or stress of their day before they can attempt to "let go" physically, mentally or otherwise. The yang flow allows this transition to occur so that when the yin series begins, both the body and the mind are more open to settle into a slow pace.

Here are a few guidelines to help you capture the essence of Elemental Yin Yang Yoga:

1. Start with one gentle posture to set the tone of your practice. It might be using a block or the wall for support, a few minutes of meditation or gentle deep breathing. If you work with a certain breathing style (like sounded breath) you can experiment with this during your yang flow, but let your breathing be natural when you come to the yin postures.

2. Find an opening posture that is suggestive of what you are working towards in your final yang posture. Typically, this would be the most challenging or vigorous part of the practice after a good warm-up. For example if you plan to do a back bend at the end of your yang flow, perhaps open your session with a gentle supported fish. If you will be doing work around the hamstrings, you might start with legs up the wall for a few minutes.

The Yang Flow

As you move through your yang flow remember the focus is on warming and strengthening the body, and on entertaining new ideas about what is possible. You don't need to strain or overwork. Be playful and creative as you flow and breathe.

The Apex Pose

The end of each yang flow finishes with what I call an "apex pose". This pose is traditionally the most challenging, warming, or vigorous asana of the sequence and feautures the main elemental energy the practice is centered around. For example an Earth Yin Yang practice may include many different asanas, but will feature core work and twists throughout the session and one of these poses is likely to be the apex of the yang sequence.

The Yin Poses

Yin postures are traditionally held for 3-5 minutes per side in stillness. While yin philosophy teaches the yogi to settle in to stillness and not be caught up or distracted by mental fluctuations (boredom, irritability, fatigue) or physical discomfort there are some things to keep in mind.

While being still is important during your postures, this instruction is coupled with a sense of relaxation or ease. Pushing yourself into a posture too deeply and then holding stillness with all your might when it becomes uncomfortable, is the opposite of yin. Instead, attempt to find a depth you know you can live with for at least five minutes in every pose. As you learn more about your physical and mental comfort level, you can explore more deeply or back off as needed in your next practice.

Remember that yin doesn't demand the deepest version of a pose, it is more important to set yourself up in a reasonable expression that does not cause pain or injury and from there, let go of reacting to thoughts, feelings and physical sensations because you know you are within a safe boundary. If you are always pushing yourself too far, you will not be able to truly let go of constantly monitoring your thoughts, feelings and sensations because you will remain on alert.

Savasana

No Elemental Yin Yang practice is complete without savasana. On the low end, your savasana should be at least ten minutes. If you have the space for more, 20-30 minutes would be ideal.

To practice savasana, lie on your mat with your arms falling open and palms face up down by your side. If you have low back tension some students enjoy having a rolled up towel or blanket under the knees.

Use this time to let go of your practice completely. This is the most yin posture of all, so avoid trying to insert an extra posture into the space meant for savasana.

As a teacher I occasionally meet students that want to use the time allowed for this final yin posture to instead meditate or do an alternative pose such as legs-up-the-wall. Although these are wonderful practices and other teachers may be open to these modifications, in Elemental Yin Yang Yoga, savasana is a very important asana and should never be skimped on or skipped. For the reason why this yin asana is so important, review Metal: On the Mat (pages 93-94).

Staying Safe: A Gentle Reminder

The yoga poses and descriptions in the following section are for informational and educational purposes only. The photos shown are to help you, the reader have a visual reference for the themes and ideas shared and are not meant to replace working with a qualified yoga instructor.

As with any physical exercise, seek professional medical advice before you attempt any poses, postures or routines in this, or any other book or source.

Yoga is meant to help you on the path of health and well-being so never push yourself to the point where you feel unwell or experience pain.

> **Get Free Videos, Audios and Elemental Resources**
> **Visit: www.aquinyoga.com/elemental**

Water Poses

While Water is one of the most yin of all the elements, it holds important themes and postures useful in the yang flow. "Flowing" itself is a watery concept and in a yoga practice that features this element the yogi would move as though she were literally transitioning between poses while standing in water.

If you have never practiced this way, as an experiment you might start with a movement like lifting your arms overhead. When you do this normally, you raise the arms without any external resistance. If however you stand in a pool with your arms down by your side, when you lift them you will notice you have to push against the "thickness" of the water to get your arms up. Conducting your entire flow with this gentle resistance can add a profound layer to your practice and help you to move with strength and grace.

Using Your Resources Wisely

Yoga can be many things, but when it comes to the Water element it is a practice of both cultivation of qi and intelligent output of qi. While the yin postures are a major player in nourishing the yogi the yang postures offer the opportunity to experiment with how much of our inner resources are required in any given situation. For more see Water: On the Mat (pages: 32-33).

Yang Poses - The Prep Work

Water yang postures are not confined to one category of pose in particular, but typically they are postures that are preparatory to master advanced asana. Downward Dog is an example of a prep pose that lends its wisdom to many other postures. Some teachers won't let their students attempt arm balances like crow or handstand until they can hold Downward Dog for at least five minutes. The advanced arm balance is something that takes time to build up to and the Water element is key in teaching the yogi how to build the strength and confidence to cross the threshold of the unknown and lift off the ground.

Downward Dog

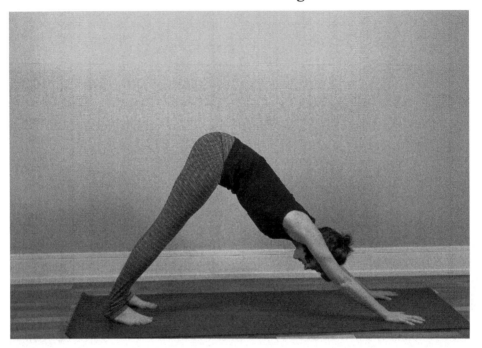

Keys:

- Stimulates qi flow through the Bladder meridian (a complex primary meridian that traverses the length of the back of the body)

- Provides a foundation for many advanced poses

Downward Dog is a staple posture in flow yoga practices. As such it is a wonderful opportunity for the yogi to check in with the body from day to day. A few moments in downward dog provides information on how the breath is moving and how the body is feeling overall. From here the yogi can make adjustments to their overall approach on the mat to suit the energy they have and the state of the body.

Twisted Star

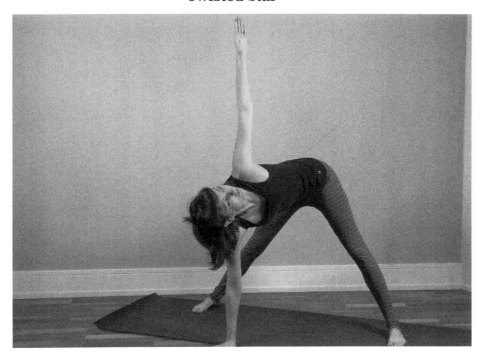

Keys:

- Stimulates qi through the Kidney meridian along the inner legs and front of the torso

- A more gentle preparatory pose for deeper folds and twists that may come later in the practice

While this posture is a twist and can be used in an Earth yang sequence, the lengthening of the torso against gravity and stretching of the legs is effective in helping qi flow through both the Kidney and Bladder meridians. For some this is a more accessible twist than deeper variations found in the average yang flow.

Water Apex - Crow

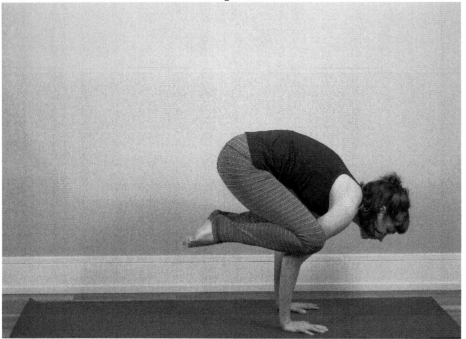

Keys:

- Uses complex movements and strength across the whole body

- Makes use of prep poses and requires facing your fear

Any posture that brings up fear could be considered a Water posture because that is the emotion of this element. Arm balances requires use of the yogis strength and the inner resolve it takes to move into the unknown and find wisdom on the other side.

Fear in arm balances is common and real. Unless you have spent time walking on your hands since you were a young child, the prospect of trusting your entire body's weight to the arms may not sound appealing.

Crow, handstand or any other posture like it requires years of prep work and an inner knowing that you have the strength, vitality, and personal resources to approach the asana. When working on a Water apex posture, you may seek out experience and expertise of other yogis who have done it. However, it is only when you are willing to do the work and cross the threshold of the unknown, into uncharted waters that you gain inner wisdom for yourself.

Be Aware: Arm balances and other Water apex poses take time and strength. Don't overdo your work around these postures. Seek out the supervision and help of a qualified teacher or movement coach to help you attempt this safely and intelligently.

Water Yin Poses

Yin postures are traditionally held for 3-5 minutes per side, in still-ness. Since the Water element is very close in nature to yin energy, these poses should be full of ease. Move into each asana only to the degree that feels reasonable and comfortable so you can relax deeply and not be distracted by physical discomfort, thoughts or feelings.

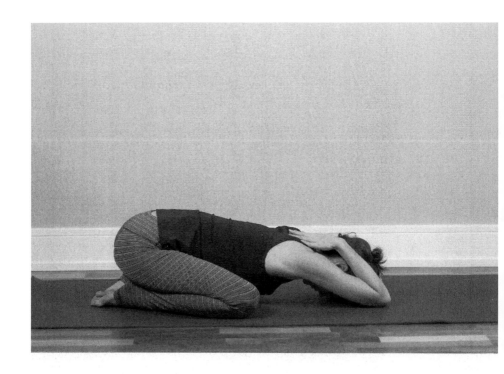

Childs Pose

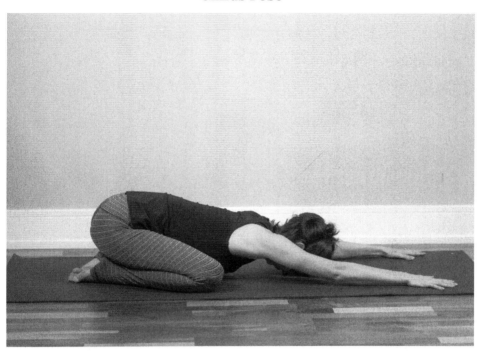

Keys:

- Turns attention inward

- Resembles the position of a fetus in the womb

Childs pose was named because of its resemblance to a fetus in the womb. Since Water energy deals directly with the yogi's Congenital Qi, resources and development, this posture connects us to early life and the source of vitality.

The pose is taken face down in an effort to turn attention inward, and away from the world.

Supported Forward Fold

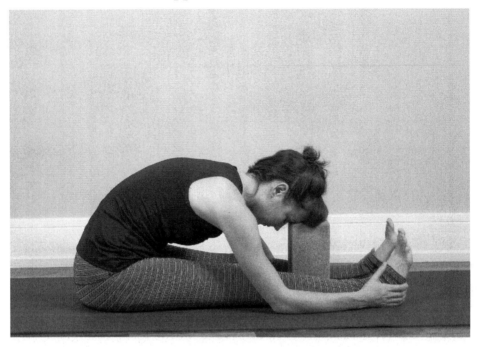

Keys:

- Invites gentle flow of qi throughout the Kidney and Bladder meridians

- Supported to allow deep release

In this gentle forward fold the yogi places the forehead on a block or the arms and moves into the posture to a gentle depth. The support of the block or the arms allows the muscles in the back a chance to soften and some yogis report when resting the forehead in this way they feel tension devolve in the face and neck.

Fire Poses

Fire is the most yang of the Five Elements. During a Fire yang flow, vigorous chest opening postures and warming backbends are featured asanas. The yin sequence may focus on gentle versions of "heart opening" poses and reminds the yogi of the connection and love all around us. The four meridians of the Fire element travel along the arms so any posture that opens or strengthens the arms can influence Fire energy.

Fire Yang - Expansion and Boundaries

The wisdom of the Fire element on the yoga mat is that it allows the yogi to expand beyond self-imposed mental restrictions. Fire yang is an opportunity to rejoice in your ability to work with the body and experiment with postures and perspectives you may believe are "out of your league".

At the same time, healthy Fire on the mat encourages you to work within reasonable, mature boundaries so that you maintain a safe and healthy practice. For example someone who has practiced yoga for several years and has a strong and healthy body may be ready to expand their repertoire of poses towards a backbend like camel. However, it would be irresponsible for a brand new student to jump into this pose without the necessary ingredients in place.

Exalted Warrior

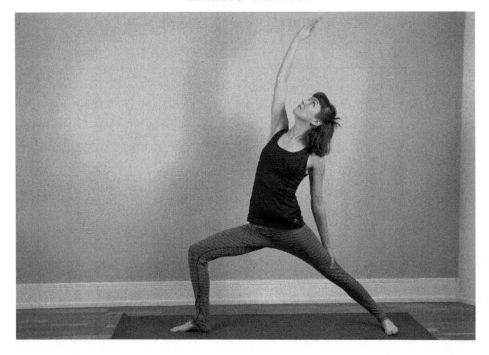

Keys:

- Stimulates qi flow along the Fire meridians

- Warming backbend with grounded legs

One meaning of the word "exalted" is to be extremely happy. This posture is a physical expression of the the emotion of Fire, joy. The joyful warrior reaching upward into a slight backbend, opening to the sky. This pose should be lighthearted and full of breath as energy courses through the body.

Dancer Pose

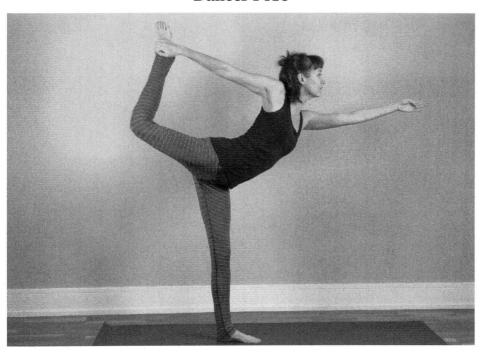

Keys:

- Warming backbend that engages the legs in preparation for other similar poses
- Conscious lifting of the chest helps to counter rounding forward

Dancer is one part backbend, one part balance. Working with this pose, the yogi learns to engage the legs and glutes in order to support the body. This posture also helps to counter hunching forward through the shoulders and upper back that has become habit for many people who work desk jobs or sit in chairs for most of the day. This posture that can inspire a lifting of your mood as you breath deep and enjoy your own expansion.

Fire Apex - Camel

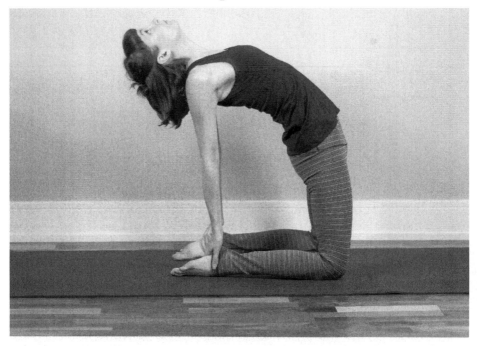

Keys:

- Grounding backbend

- Use of the arms and opening of chest stimulates qi flow in Fire meridians

Camel is a Fire apex pose that can bring up a number of responses in yogis. For some it is a beautiful and empowering backbend. For others it is frustrating and may trigger feelings of anxiety. In order to sustain this posture the yogi must be fully connected from head to toe, simultaneously trusting their strength and respecting mental and physical boundaries.

Similar to the emotion and themes of Fire, joy and expansion are wonderful but only when rooted in reality. Camel pose offers the opportunity to both open the heart and remain grounded.

Be Aware: Active legs are key to the safety of this posture. Go back slowly and deliberately without twisting your spine or losing the connection to your legs.

Fire Yin Poses

Fire yin poses should be used sparingly if the main focus of the practice has been on backbends and chest openers. Keeping with the themes of both expansion and maintaining healthy boundaries on the mat, too much backbending can be draining. Fire yin poses are a wonderful counter to other elements when used gently and should never be held if you experience pain.

Melting Heart Pose

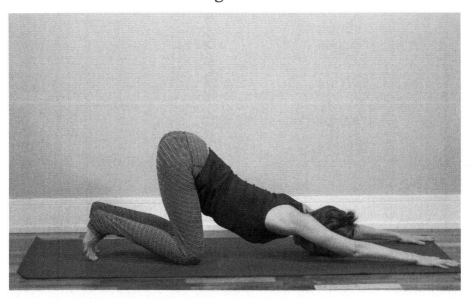

Key:
  • Similar to Child's Pose with a backbend

In this pose the hips are stacked over the knees and the chest is lengthened on to the mat or supported by a bolster. The arms reach forward allowing qi to flow through the Fire meridians.

Sphinx Pose

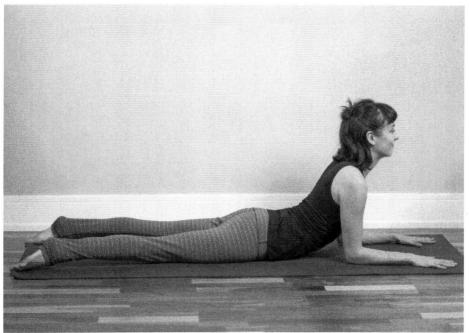

Keys:

- A gentle backbend that is easier to hold than most

Sphinx pose is one of the more accessible backbends of yoga. The legs and pelvis are grounded with little effort and the lifting of the chest is supported passively by the position of the arms. Unlike most backbends which can't be sustained for extended periods of time, sphinx is yin in nature as it doesn't require a constant output of energy.

Wood Poses

Wood energy on the yoga mat can be found in the foundation and focus of the yang flow and the freedom of letting go in the yin poses. Wood postures, both yin and yang, offer the opportunity to encounter irritability and frustration in a controlled environment.

Wood Yang Poses

Wood yang asanas require a generous amount of effort and, over time, even the strongest yogi will need to come out of the posture when it becomes too much. This is not a problem, but at that moment it is helpful to observe the conclusion you are drawing or the response you are having.

Do you notice yourself stuck on feelings of failure or anger if you couldn't sustain the posture?
If you tend to feel inner anger (wood's emotion) or frustration, consider that your experience is merely another expression of energy and it is self-generated. Stress and anger only come up when you make a story about the moments you are stringing together. "My arms are shaking" may be a fact, but "I'm too weak for this pose and my teacher is mean for making me do it", is a story you are creating.

That story turns into a belief and that belief actually takes away the energy you need to do the pose you're trying to do in the first place. Use the energy of the Wood element not only to help keep you from getting stuck on negative beliefs you hold but to grow and deepen your practice.

Tree Pose

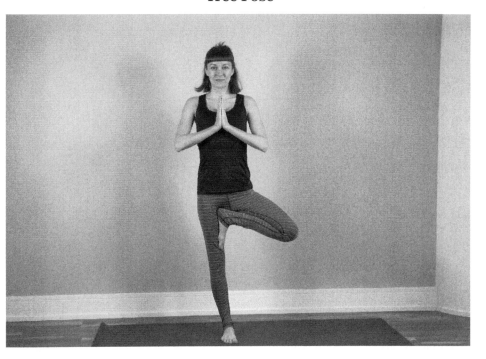

Keys:

- Requires both a solid foundation and flexibility

- Strengthens the ankles and feet near the Wood meridians

Tree pose is wood down to its very name. Balance postures require a solid foundation, focused awareness and enough flexibility to blow in the wind. If the yogi is missing any one piece, the tree will not be stable and they will have the opportunity to see their response in the face of struggling to hold the pose. This asana is particularly strengthening to the ankle in areas that the Liver and Gall Bladder channel pass through.

Warrior 1

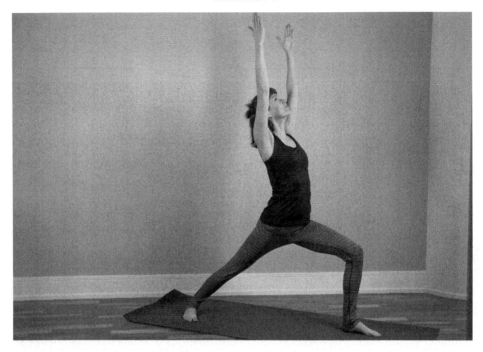

Keys:

- Deeply grounded legs with upward reaching torso

- Stimulates qi flow to Wood meridians

Warrior 1 is a pose that mimics the themes of Wood beautifully. The legs are grounded and provide a solid foundation for the torso to rest upon. The torso focuses energy upwards through the reaching arms. This posture moves qi through the meandering paths of the Liver and Gall Bladder meridians along the legs and side of the body.

Wood Apex - Plank Sequence

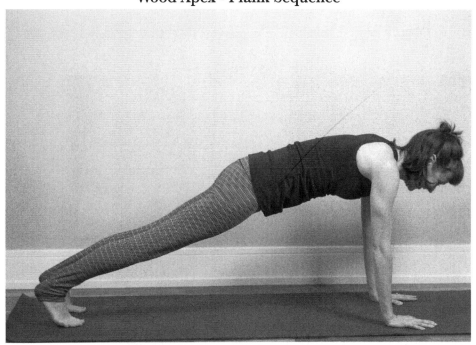

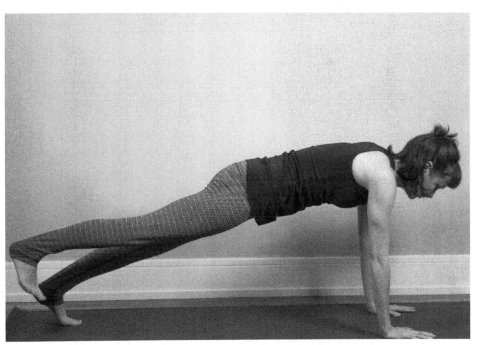

Keys:

- strong legs and core required

- the Wood meridians travel along the side of the body and legs and this areas is deeply engaged

Plank poses and their variations require full body participation in order to be sustained beyond a few breaths. In this Wood yang posture the midsection and legs (which host a portion of the Liver and Gall Bladder meridians) are engaged.

To make this a more active sequence the yogi can practice slowly lifting the legs one at a time without moving the hips up and down. Build up to as many repetitions as you can while maintaining a steady breath and connection throughout the body.

Be Aware: This sequence requires tremendous arm, leg and core strength. To modify you may wish to keep one knee on the mat or work from the elbows and allow the pose to strengthen over time.

Wood Yin Poses

Although still yin in nature, Wood yin poses tend to be challenging compared to other elements. These asanas may require some effort to stay in the posture. The instructions are the same; get into the pose to a reasonable degree, allow stillness, relaxation and let go of needing to respond to any physical, emotional or mental fluctuations that arise.

Gate Pose

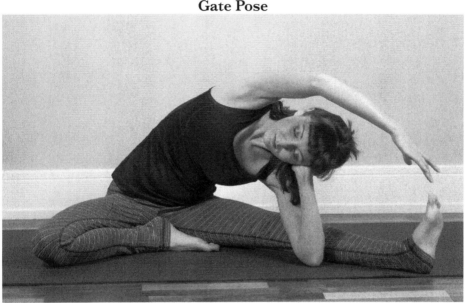

Keys:

- grounded side bend

- support for the head and neck helps to ease tension

Side bending is underused in most forms of yoga. Holding a yin pose like this for a few minutes can ease tension along the waist and low back. Resting the head on the hand gives the neck a chance to release. The yogi may also wrap the top arm behind the back for more support and depth instead of letting it hang in space.

Resting Lunge

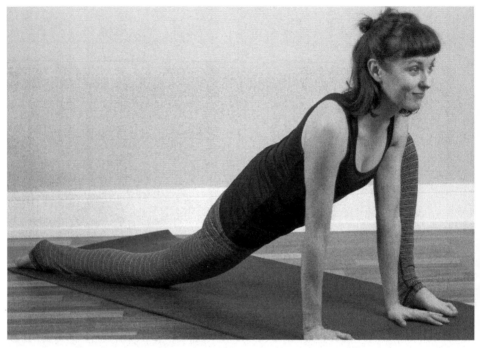

Keys:

- Find an appropriate depth in order to hold the pose in stillness

- Deep hip, quad, hamstring stretch

Resting lunge may not feel as relaxing as the name suggests. Most yogis require the support of a blanket under the back knee or thigh and possibly blocks under the hands to find depth that is appropriate. Although this is a yin pose, if the yogi goes too far, they will experience tension and frustration trying to hold it for the full 3-5 minutes on each side.

As always, the deepest version of the pose is not the most yin. Find a way of being in the pose you can live with comfortably for the duration of the yin cycle.

Metal Poses

Metal postures are similar to Fire poses because they typically open the chest and some backbends may be included. However, the connection with the Lungs and Large Intestine (taking in and letting go) makes these postures more yin in nature than Fire's variations.

Metal Yang Poses

In a Metal yang flow many standing postures may be used but poses that feature solid spreading arms are specifically useful because the Metal meridians (Lung and Large Intestine) stretch along the top and bottom of the radial line of the arm (the thumb-side) before meeting the torso. Attention to steady breathing is also key to the metal nature of these poses.

While typically, holding a posture is considered yin, holding a very active posture like Warrior 2, Triangle or Side Plank requires the patience of a warrior. A good warrior waits for the right moment to act and can wait all day because she is in a state of emptiness. The warrior does not hold themselves taut like a bowstring while waiting to strike, but relaxes into position, knowing that her energy is valuable and should not be wasted or exerted in the frenzy of anticipation.

In Metal yang postures the yogi is ready, alert and responds only to the situation he is in. He does not race to get to the next moment, but stays with dignity and grace in the present.

Warrior 2

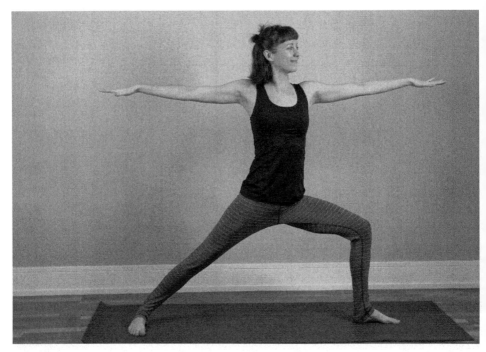

Keys:

- Opening and strengthening of the arms stimulates qi flow through the Lung and Large Intestine meridians

- A long hold takes patience and emptiness

In a Metal yang flow any of the warrior postures can be used. Warrior 2 in particular has a focus on opening the front of the body and reaching the inner arms long and strong. If the yogi holds unnecessary tension they will tire and the dignity of the pose will be lost.

Metal Apex - Side Plank

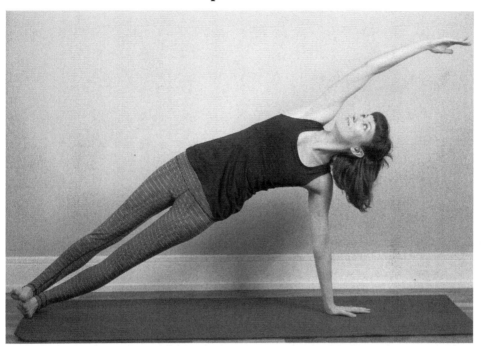

Key:

- Requires strength, stability, patience and breath

While planks fit nicely with several elements (Wood and Water) a side plank is useful as a Metal apex posture. In this version the emphasis is on reaching the arm overhead and stimulating the Metal meridians along the radial line and up the side of the arm, the front of the shoulder and chest.

Be Aware: This posture takes a great deal of strength. Some yogis prefer to do this pose with a knee and a elbow on the ground as a support instead of keeping the bottom arm and leg straight. As with any posture, find an alternative posture that suits you best and do not push through pain or injury.

Triangle

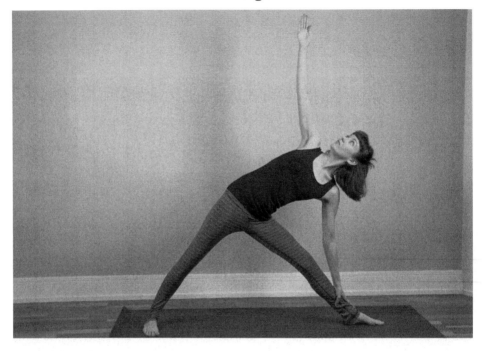

Keys:

- Opening of the arms stimulates flow through the Metal meridians

- Side opening gives the opportunity to lift up and out of the legs and breath deeply

Energetically in triangle the intention is to lift up towards the top arm and open the chest instead of sinking down into the legs. This posture holds several complex actions at once depending on the school of alignment you come from. As such it is easy to loose one of the fundamental pillars of practice, the breath. In an attempt to go deeper into the pose the yogi may lose their breath connection and not know whether the posture is effective or has gone too far to retain its value.

Metal Yin Poses

Of all the elements, Metal is one of the most yin. The deepest yin pose of all is Savasana but there are other gentle poses that encourage the yogi to let go deeply and spend time free doing nothing at all. Metal yin poses typically require the support of props like yoga blocks, bolsters or a thick blanket. If those items are not available you can substitute these poses with a few minutes of witnessing your breath.

It is difficult to observe the breath without judgment or trying to change it but spending five to ten minutes giving your attention to a process that supports life can be a beautiful transition into savasana to complete your practice.

If you have a preferred pranayama (breath and energy work) practice you might also use this to cultivate "Metal" energy.

Keep in mind that vigorous pranayama that builds heat belongs in the yang portion of class and breathwork that is soothing and inspires you to let go is more yin in nature.

Supported Fish

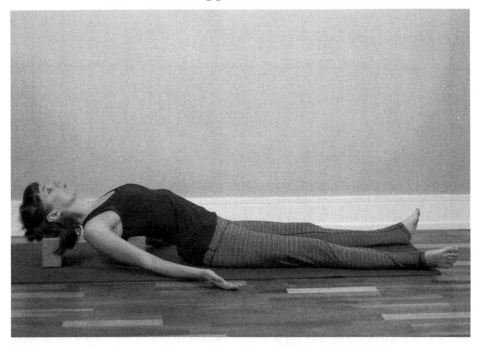

Keys:

- Gentle chest opener

- Opening the arms provides space for qi and blood to flow through Metal meridians

Fish pose has several mythological tales surrounding it. One is of a fish that went swimming by a sage giving a teaching. The fish was so enraptured with the yogic wisdom being taught that he popped his head out of the water in order to absorb the energy and mysteries being explored.

In supported fish, one block is placed under the head and the other is placed under heart-centre at the same height. The arms move away from the body for a light stretch across the chest and arms.

Spinal Roll

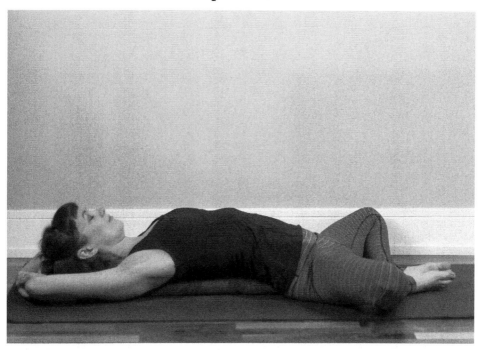

Keys:

- A thick blanket under the length of the spine creates an opening

- Support allows the yogi to rest here for a full yin cycle comfortably

Although at first glance you may not notice it in the image, there is a rolled up blanket that is supporting the length of the spine. As a Metal yin pose, the soles of the feet together, knees wide along with the arms overhead provide a body-wide, graceful letting go. This is a lovely pose to begin a yoga practice with or to take just before savasana.

Earth Poses

Twists and "core work" are the main types of Earth yang postures because they focus on strength and movement through the centre of the body. The Earth element has a strong connection to digestion and the muscles that sytem helps to build. However, when it comes to "core work" the intent isn't to carve out a six-pack of abs that many fitness enthusiasts chase in their workouts.

The yoga relationship with these types of postures is to strengthen the centre of the body. This is more than simply the abdominal muscles but also the support and stabilization muscles of the torso.

Earth Yang & The Belly

Many people hold tension in the belly due to stress in their daily lives. One benefit of twists and core work is that rather than unconsciously tensing the belly the way much of the world does, we learn to engage our muscles mindfully and strengthen them. Since the Earth element has a relationship with rumination and overthinking it makes sense that working with this element offers tools of support to counter the negative effects of holding tension in the belly.

The best moment of a core sequence or twist is the often the moment it is over. There is a satisfaction knowing you have used your energetic potential for a concentrated burst of energy and the torso (and belly especially) can finally relax and receive the qi and blood flowing without stress or strain blocking the path.

Twisted Squat

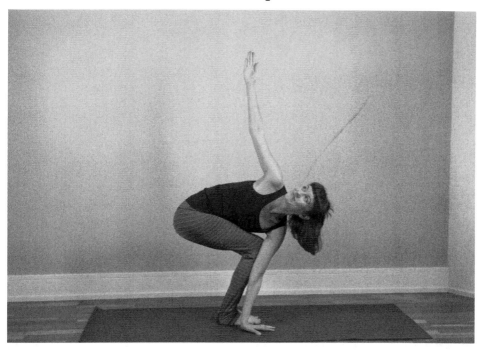

Keys:

- deep twist with active muscular engagement

- stimulates qi flow along Spleen and Stomach meridians

While any posture that both strengthens and twists can be Earth in nature, this posture is a great example. Essentially a twisting squat the focus of this pose is on the centre of the body and the digestive organs.

This Earth yang asana warms the body and activates many areas along the both the Spleen and Stomach meridians (especially stimulating for the quads and several Stomach channel areas).

Revolved Side Angle

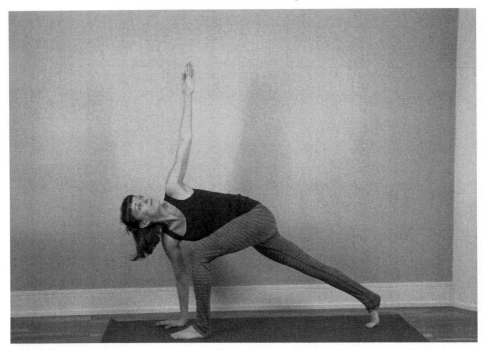

Keys:

- warming twist with active muscle engagement (muscles are the tissues that represent the Earth element)

- stimulates qi flow along Spleen and Stomach meridians

This combination of twist and lunge not only activates the Earth meridians through the torso and legs but it helps the yogi lengthen into the twist rather than hunch forward.

This Earth yang asana warms several muscles groups while strengthening the body.

Earth Apex - Reclined Core Work

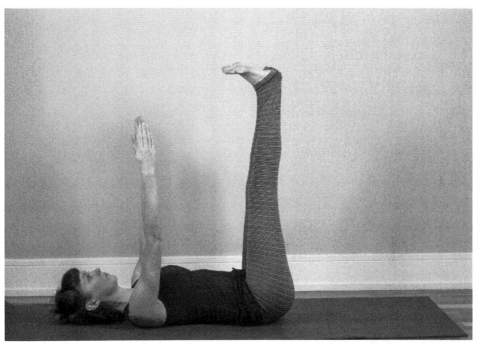

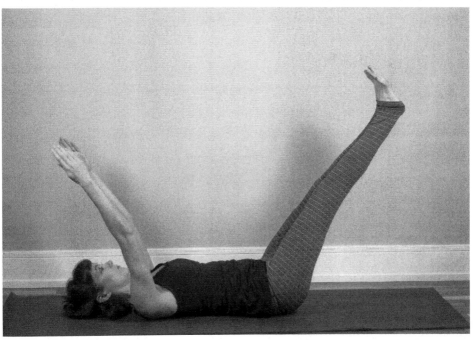

Keys:

- strengthen and stabilize the torso to support the limbs and all manner of movement

- stimulates qi and blood flow especially through the Stomach channel along the front of the torso over the abdominal muscles

As an apex posture a simple core sequence might involve starting with the abdomen strongly braced. The arms stack over the shoulders and heels stack over the hips. Slowly and with control, the legs are lowered down towards the floor and the arms overhead. The arms and legs should only be lowered to the degree that the yogi feels they have control and can lift or lower the limbs smoothly. This movement is graceful without swinging the arms and legs.

Be Aware: If the back feels sore or weak the legs should not be lowered as far and the knees may be bent. If the back is still unhappy, find a different posture instead.

Earth Yin Poses

The postures that best represent yin for the Earth element are twists that require as little effort as possible. Although there are deeper ways to twist even when lying on the floor, a yin twist is one that could be held easily for several minutes without tension. Earth yin poses are very similar to restorative yoga and props are always welcome to support the yogi.

Reclined Twist

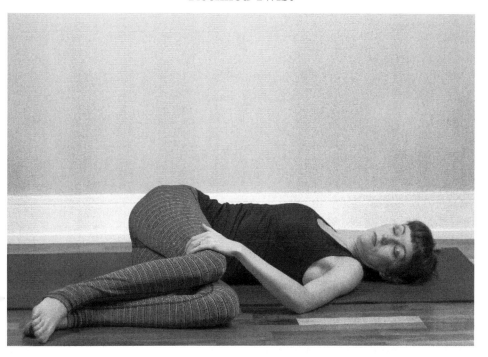

Keys:

- An extremely nourishing twist

- Moves qi and blood through side body Earth meridians

Many yogis find this to be among the most nourishing and relaxing of all yin postures. Fully supported by the ground below and held by gravity above, this asana is nourishing for the mind and body. For additional support place a block between your knees to ease pressure from the hips and low back.

Stag Twist

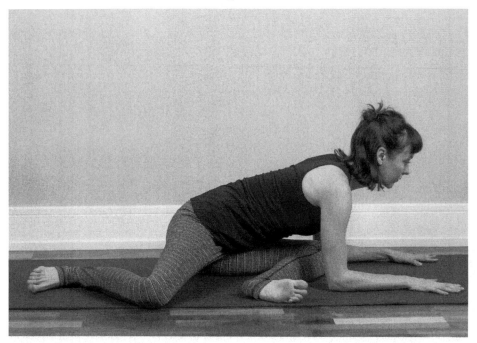

Keys:

- Gentle twist

- Resting here helps qi and blood flow easily move through the Earth meridians

The pose begins by taking the legs into an "L" shape or 90 degree angle and then bending the knees and adjusting the hips for comfort. Slowly the yogi twists towards the front leg and if available comes down towards the elbows. There is a gentle "wringing" out of the abdomen that happens naturally with the breath and the Earth meridians receive what they need.

Final Pose - Savasana

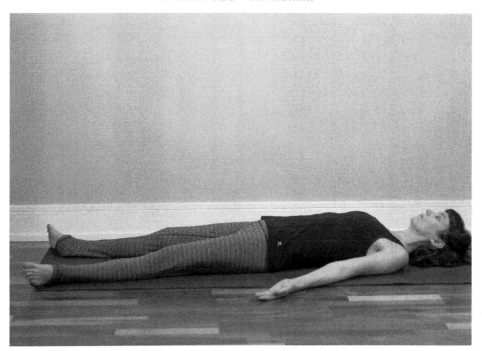

Key:

- Final letting go

- Apex of the yin sequence

Savasana is the final letting go at the end of a session. For more on the philosophy and importance of this pose read the Metal theory chapter.

Get Free Videos, Audios and Elemental Resources
Visit: www.aquinyoga.com/elemental

Sample Elemental Yin Yang Practice

Theme: Earth
- being supported
- yin and yang self-care

Opening
5 minutes of meditation

Yang Flow
Sun Salutations
Warrior 2
Revolved Side angle
Triangle
Twisted Star
Warrior 1
Twisted Squat
Reclined Core Work

Yin
Stag Twist
Spinal Roll
Childs pose
Reclined twist

Savasana

Resources and Further Reading

Yin Yang Yoga Book Free Extras
http://www.aquinyoga.com/elemental

Build a Yin Yang Home Practice
https://www.udemy.com/yin-yang-yoga-build-your-home-practice/

Teach Yin Yang Yoga
http://www.aquinyoga.com/yin-yang-ytt

Books on Chinese Medicine
In the last decade I from many practitioners in school and through incredible books. When it came time to write this book there were a few resources I returned to frequently. Although all are meant for Chinese Medicine practitioners, each can shed light and depth on the way of thinking that helped birth Elemental Yin Yang Yoga.

Nourishing Destiny: The Inner Tradition of Chinese Medicine - Lonny Jarrett

Five Spirits: Alchemical Acupuncture for Psychological and Spiritual Healing - Lorie Dechar

The Web That Has No Weaver - Ted Kaptchuk

The Foundations of Chinese Medicine: A Comprehensive Text - Giovanni Maciocia

The Medical Classic of the Yellow Emperor - Zhu Ming

Printed in Great Britain
by Amazon

81945808R00104